Tuning Fork Therapy®

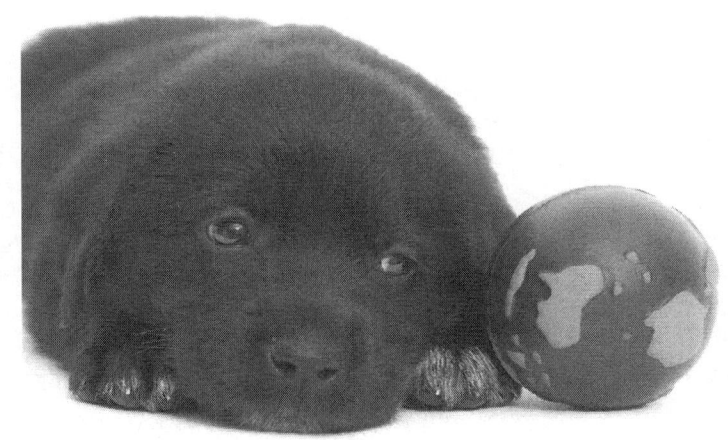

Using Tuning Forks on Dogs Acupuncture Points

Francine Milford

Tuning Fork Therapy® using Tuning Forks on Dogs
Acupuncture Points by Francine Milford

First Edition 2008, Revised Edition 2012

ISBN: 978-1-4357-4031-0

Photographs and Illustrations by Francine Milford

The techniques, ideas, and suggestions presented in this book
are not intended as a substitute for proper medical advice.
Any application of the techniques, ideas, and suggestions in
this book is at the reader's sole discretion and risk.

Table of Contents

Chapter One..**5**

   Introduction to Tuning Fork Therapy®.........................5

   The Science of Sound 6

   The Nature of Sound Waves.....................................7

   What are Harmonics?...8

   Pitch...10

   Nature of Frequency...11

Chapter Two..**15**

   Hearing and the Canine Ear.....................................15

Chapter Three...**19**

   The Dog's Ear..19

Chapter Four..**27**

   History of the Tuning Fork.......................................27

Chapter Five...**31**

   The Tuning Fork..31

Chapter Six..**41**

   Elements and Tuning Forks......................................41

     The 'C' Tuning Fork (Middle/Low)...........................43

     The 'D' Tuning Fork...44

     The 'E' Tuning Fork...45

     The 'F' Tuning Fork...46

     The 'G' Tuning Fork...47

     The 'A' Tuning Fork...48

     The 'B' Tuning Fork...49

Chapter Seven…………………………………………………**51**

    What is Acupuncture…………………………………...51

Chapter Eight.…..**59**

    Acupuncture/Sound Session……………………………59

Chapter Nine.………………………………………….…..**69**

    10 Acupuncture points for Sound Healing……………69

    10 Major points..73

    Point#1...77

    Point#2...78

    Point#3...80

    Point#4...82

    Point#5...84

    Point#6...85

    Point#7...86

    Point#8...88

    Point#9...90

    Point#10..92

Chapter Nine...**69**

    Ways to Select your Tuning Forks………………...69

    Methods and Techniques...................................97

    Spiral Technique...98

    Horizontal Technique......................................99

    Aura Smoothing Technique...............................101

    Tuning Fork Therapy® session for your pet………...103

About the Author....**107**

References...**111**

Chapter One

Introduction to Tuning Fork Therapy®

The Science of Sound

All around us are forces of energy. The air we breathe, the water we drink, and the foods we eat are all forces of energy. So, too, are the sounds we hear. A bird sings, a frog croaks, a bell rings...all these sounds and more elicit a specific response in our minds. Whether we are aware of it or not we are subconsciously taking note and filing away information about the world around us.

In our daily lives, we are inundated with a variety of sounds. For the most part, we have trained ourselves to filter out the "noise" of day-to-day living in a modern society. A case in point, how many passing cars do you now single out and count in a day? For the most part you have only made yourself aware that there are passing cars and never give them another notice unless something unexpected happens, such as a crash.

Have you ever noticed how your attention turns to the sound of an automobile crash? For those of you who are parents, even the sound a child calling for its mother can grab your attention.

This is the world we live in, the world of sound communication.

The study of sound includes knowledge of sound waves, compression waves and mechanical waves. I have taken this time to break the study down into easy to understand components.

It is my wish that you receive a basic understanding of how sound travels and is received. There are many good books on the market for those of you who wish to devote more time in the study of sound. For you, I encourage you to continue your studies.

We will begin our study with the sound wave. A sound wave in Tuning Fork Therapy® is created by striking one tuning fork against another surface. This surface can be another tuning fork, the palm of your hand or a tuning fork activator.

What a sound wave needs most is matter through which to travel. Matter can be anything including air, water, metals, even a wall-but sound cannot pass through a vacuum.

A popular classroom experiment to prove this point; a teacher will place a bell in a sealed, see-through ball. You can watch the bell as it is being rung, but you will hear no sound. A bell that is rung in a vacuum makes no sound at all.

We can take this knowledge of sound passing through objects to the use of tuning forks on our own bodies. Because our bodies are solid, sound waves can pass through our skin, organs, tissues, right down to the very cells of our bodies.

The development of Tuning Fork Therapy® is based on my belief that as sound waves pass through the body, they elicit responses within the body's systems. These systems in turn, react to the sound waves and vibrations and are restored to a healthier and more harmonic base.

Within this course, I have presented information on how certain sounds and vibrations affect specific areas of the body. There have been some remarkable studies on how various cells, especially cancer cells, respond to sound waves.

This is a new frontier and we are just beginning to understand how sound waves can be used to help heal our body, mind, and spirit.

As more practitioners begin incorporating tuning forks and sound therapy into their practices, more information will be developed and shared in this exciting field. I look forward to hearing about your own experiences while using Tuning Fork Therapy® in your own practice.

I encourage you visit the many science and physics websites that are on the Internet and watch for yourself how sound is measured and captured on film. These films make for exciting and informative viewings.

The Nature of Sound Waves

Sounds are all around us and yet we seldom take the time to discover each characteristic. Have you ever wondered how a sound is created and received by our ears?

Sound waves are created when objects vibrate through a medium (i.e. water, air, bones, or metal) from one location to another. One such medium that we will use through this book is the human body.

A tuning fork is a metal object that has one handle and two tines. The two tines vibrate when they are struck against another object, whether that object is your hand, rubber mallet, or another tuning fork.

When struck, the tines of the tuning fork begin to vibrate back and forth. This vibrating begins to disturb the air molecules that surround the tuning fork and, like a ripple in the water, these air molecules begin to disturb the air molecules next to them creating the Slinky effect.

It is the motion of this air molecule disturbance coming from the tuning fork that is called a sound wave. We know the tuning fork is vibrating because we can hear it. Since the tines of the tuning fork are vibrating at a very high frequency, we cannot actually see movement.

In the case of tuning forks, sound is measured in movement or vibrations. This movement is referred to as Hertz or Hz for short and was named for the man who invented the term, Heninrich Rudolph Hertz and represents one vibration per second.

The number listed on each of the tuning forks is in Hz and correlates to the rate of vibrations per second that the tuning fork is associated with. The lower the number listed on the tuning fork, the slower the vibrations per second.

See the diagram on the next page for clarification.

A Tuning Fork vibrating 1 time each second would have a frequency of 1 Hz.

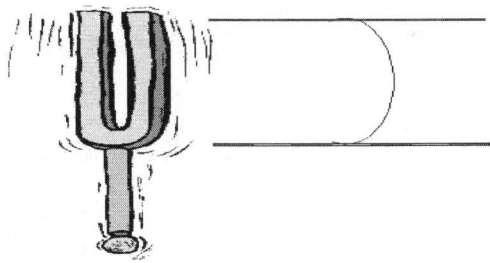

A Tuning Fork vibrating 5 times each second would have a frequency of 5 Hz,

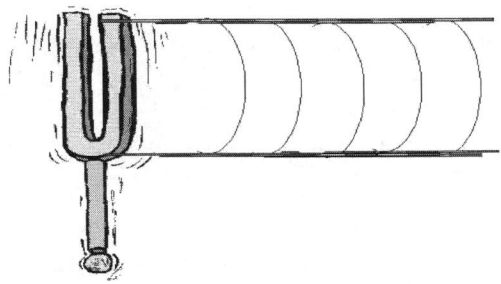

When the tuning fork is being used to correspond to the Middle C on the piano, then the tines of the tuning fork are said to be vibrating at a frequency of 256 HZ (that's 256 vibrations per second). Likewise, a tuning fork listed as 512 HZ will vibrate at 512 vibrations per second—two times the frequency of the tuning fork.

What are Harmonics?

Harmonics are what enable you to hear a sound and recognize what instrument played it. They enable you to tell the difference between a C note being played on a piano, and a C note being played on a flute. Even though instruments have the same fundamental frequency and pitch, they have a different proportional mix of harmonics that we call timbre.

Our own voice consists of distinct measures of harmonics. This is how we can distinguish familiar voices. The sounds we hear contain many different frequencies. When we listen closely to a sound, we are actually hearing a composite of different pitches. The brain distinguishes these sound sources based on specific relationships between those pitches. A sound's "spectrum" is the sound's total collection of pitches and their relative strengths.

Each harmonic spectrum consists of a fundamental tone and a number of overtones that are spaced according to the harmonic overtone series. For example, if the fundamental tone is 100 Hz (100 cycles per second), the overtones will be 200 Hz, 300 Hz, 400 Hz, etc. The timbre of the sound is determined by the strength of the different overtones. Each musical instrument has its own timbre. The more complicated the sound, the more involved the spectrums. The timbre may also change over time.

High and Low Frequency

Even though we know a tuning fork is vibrating because we can hear the sound that it is making, we cannot always see the tines themselves vibrating.

When struck, or activated, the tines of the tuning forks move back and forth at a frequency that corresponds to the Hertz of the tuning fork.

So, a tuning fork with a Hertz of 256 will vibrate at a slower rate than a tuning fork with a Hertz of 512. The lower the Hertz, the slower is the rate of vibration and the better are your chances of seeing the tines of the tuning fork move.

Frequencies can be divided up into low and high frequencies. In the example above, the tuning fork at 256 Hz would be considered a low frequency and the tuning fork at 512 Hz would be considered a high frequency.

The normal range of hearing for humans is approximately 20 Hz to 20,000 Hz. Frequencies below 20 Hz are called *infrasound* and frequencies above 20,000 Hz are called *ultrasound*.

This is how frequency is measured in graph form:

300 Hz – Low frequency

Time

Period

500 Hz – High frequency

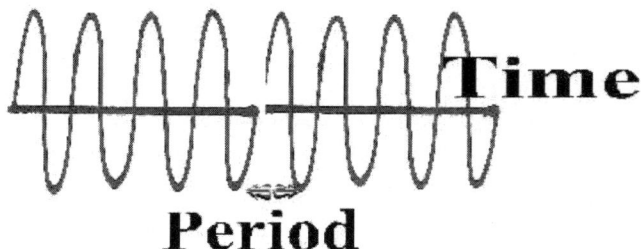

Period

Pitch

Pitch is the sensation of a frequency. A high pitch sound will correlate to a high frequency sound wave. Likewise, a low pitch sound will correlate to a low frequency sound wave.

Many musicians and singers can tell the slightest of differences between a pitch of two sounds that are within 2 Hz of each other.

Compression Waves

Sound waves are also called compression waves. To illustrate what a compression wave looks like, you need to use a Slinky toy. It is best to have two people perform this experiment. One person will hold one end of the Slinky while the other person will hold the opposite end. There should be some tension in the spring but it should not droop.

Now, one person will grab several coils of the Slinky and then release them. What you will notice is that the coils will immediately go across to the other end of the Slinky, and then return to the person who released them in the first place. This creates a sort of yo-yo affect.

This handful of coils will stay together as they travel back and forth. Sound waves travel together in much the same way. In sound waves, compressions are areas where the air particles, like the rings of the Slinky, are compressed together.

The opposite of Compression is Rarefaction. Compressions are regions of high air pressure where air particles are compressed, while Rarefactions are regions of low air pressure where air particles are spread apart. For this reason, sound waves are also known as pressure waves; a sound wave creates a repeating pattern of high-pressure (Compression) and low-pressure (Rarefaction) regions that move through a given medium.

The Nature of Frequency

Almost all objects will vibrate when they are hit or plucked. Even dropping a pencil on the floor will create a vibration, a movement of air molecules. It will also create a sound.

Each sound has its' own vibration, or natural frequency. Objects that vibrate at a single tone are called *pure tones*. An example of a pure tone would be a flute or tuba. These sounds are rich and full.

Some sounds that objects make are not pure tones in that it changes depending upon a number of circumstances. These sounds are what we call *noise*.

If you drop a lid of a pot on the floor, you will most definitely hear a complex sound wave that can called clunky or noisy. But the sound changes if you drop the lid of the pot on a carpet, or in the swimming pool.

If you activate and vibrate a tuning fork with a 512 Hz., the sound will always be constant whether you are standing in your house or outside in the park.

In determining the actual frequency at which an object will vibrate, a simple formula was devised:

Frequency = Speed/Wavelength

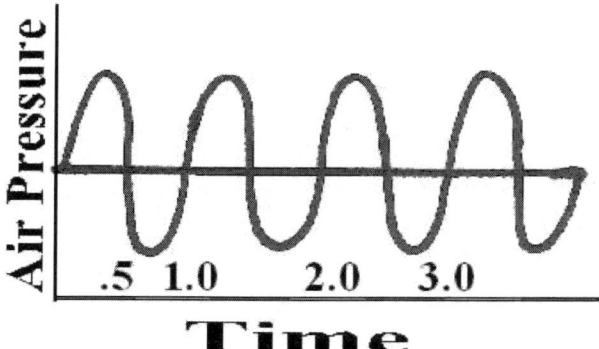

1. represents 1 cycle

Chapter Two

Hearing and the Canine Ear

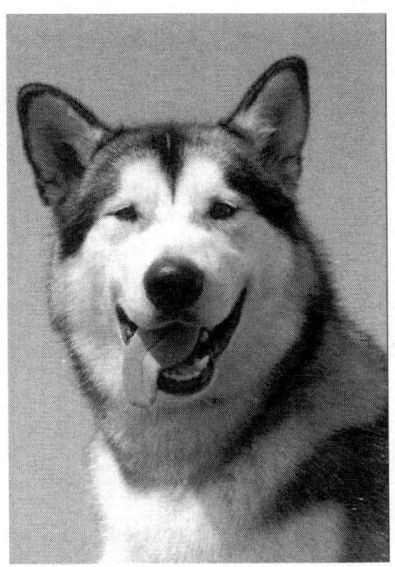

Tuning Forks and Dog's Hearing

Just like in humans, noise and sounds can affect the dog. All around the dog's environment are noises such as TVs, appliance, music, traffic, human voices, etc. Some noises, such as music that is played at high volumes for an extended period of time, can comprise the pet's immune system.

The term *'decibel'* is used to measure how loud a sound is. Dogs and cats can hear sounds at a much higher decibel than the human ear can. Remember the dog whistle? Humans can't hear the high decibel of a dog whistle-but your pet sure will. Sounds that fall into the decibel range can cause your pet pain.

Some high decibel sounds like the crack of a lightning bolt on a stormy day can send some pets running under the bed whimpering in pain. So the next time your turn your TV or stereo up on full blast, you might want to consider how this will make your pet feel.

Another term for the sound waves that we just discussed is **sound energy**. It is this sound energy that the ear picks up and converts to a mechanical energy, then to a nerve impulse. It is the nerve impulse that transmits the information to the brain.

It is through the ears' ability to accomplish this task that we are able to perceive the pitch of sounds. Through this ability to perceive different pitches we are also able to detect the sound waves' frequency, loudness, amplitude, and timbre.

For canines, they can move their ears to help them pinpoint the origin (or direction) that a sound is coming in. Like little radio dishes, a canine's ear can pick up and detect sounds at a range that is approximately four times greater than that of humans.

In addition to hearing sounds, dogs can perceive sounds by feeling the vibrations in their body. This is how many animals know that an earthquake, or some other natural disasters is about to happen. They always say, if you see animals running for high ground, you should be following them.

But all dogs do not have the same ability to hear. Some breeds are actually better at this than others. Dog breeds that have erect ears are better at hearing sounds than dog breeds that have floppy ears. And just like in humans, younger dogs have a better ability to hear than older ones do. Even with our canine friends, humans and dogs alike may lose their ability to hear as they age. And for some, deafness may just be a hereditary factor.

Some dogs may also be more sensitive to sounds than other dogs would be. For these dogs, high decibels may be more painful. For dogs with high sensitivity, the sound from a music box may bring them pain. Some dogs will bark at the sounds that they hear (even when their human owners cannot hear the sounds).

Just like some mothers would be able to pick up the sound of their crying baby in a room full of crying babies, dogs have the ability to detect a particular sound (like their owners voice) from a mixture of sounds and noises.

If you have a pet that is sensitive to sounds, then please keep them away from loud TVs, music, and events like watching fireworks on the Fourth of July. Keep your pet indoors, cover their ears, and be sure that they are receiving proper check-ups and health exams.

In addition to hearing, the ear functions as the sense organ of equilibrium and balance in the body. When stimulation activates the receptors involved with hearing and balance, this is mechanical. The receptors are called mechanoreceptors.

In the previous chapter we talked about Hertz (Hz). One Hz is 1 cycle or wave/second. We know that sound ranges from 1 Hz – 100,000 Hz. Another addition to the Hz is the abbreviation of 'k' which stands for 1,000 (kilo). Using this new abbreviation, we can say that sound reaches 100kHz (100,000Hz).

People's auditory receptors can react to sounds with frequencies ranging from 16,000 and 20,000 cycles per second. However, the optimal frequency ranges between 1,000 and 2,000 per second. Children (up until puberty) can hear higher pitch sounds than adults.

Chart of human and animal sound ability:

Human	hears 20-23 kHz
Dogs	hears up to 45 kHz
Cats	hears up to 64 kHz
Bats	hears up to 110 kHz (ultrasound)
Dolphins/Porpoises	hears up to 150 kHz (ultrasound)

What I find fascinating is how sound can travel to the brain when one is deaf. This is very interesting and to date there has not been much study on the use of tuning forks on a deaf person. In Tuning Fork Therapy®, the vibrations of the tuning fork can be just as effective as the sound one hears during the session. In this way, even deaf people can "feel" the sensations and vibrations in their bodies.

As research to support this theory, try to cover your ears with ear muffs or cotton. Now, activate a tuning fork and place the tip of the handle of the vibrating tuning fork on your body. Can you feel the vibration in your body?

Now, slowly wave the vibrating tuning fork just above your skin and see if you can sense or feel the vibration of the tuning fork. When your senses are honed, you will find it very easy to feel the tuning forks vibrating close to your body.

<u>Caution:</u>   When using tuning forks on animals, do NOT activate the tuning fork close to their ears as this may startle the animal, make them nervous, or hurt their ears.

Chapter Three

The Dog's Ear

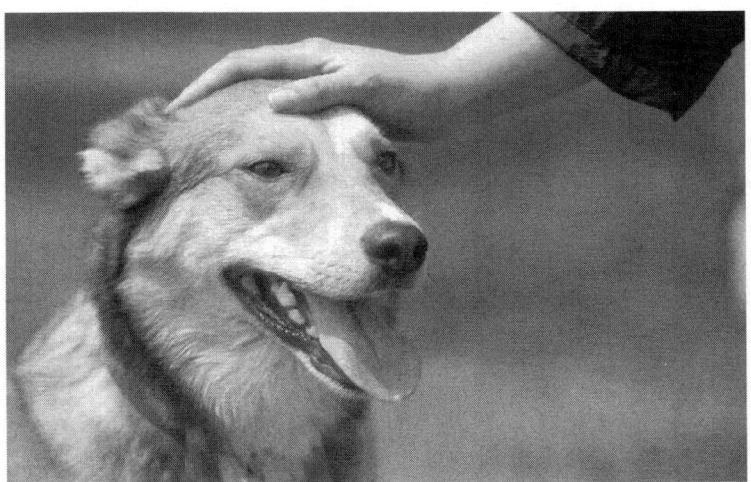

The dog's ear has more than 10 muscles that they can use to change their shape and positioning. From bending the ears to turning them nearly 180 degrees around, your pet can use their ears to express their emotions and intentions.

A dog that has their ears pulled back and is showing their teeth while growling is certainly one animal that I would not want to approach. A dog that cocks their head to one side and extends one ear straight up is a dog that has just picked up a sound that has intrigued it.

Your pet can also suffer from allergies, tumors, polyp, and ear infections-all of which can affect their hearing. If your pet has allergies, it may have trouble hearing until the allergies are cleared up.

If your pet has fluid in the middle ear from flushing, then it may take one week to 10 days before the fluid can be absorbed and hearing restored. If your pet has ear infections, especially chronic ones, then they lose the ability to hear high decibels of sound over time due to the thickening and hardening of ossicles (small bones found in the middle ear).

Tumors or polyps found in the middle ear may block the movement air, causing deafness. Perception of air movement is necessary to hear high frequency sounds. Your pet may still be able to hear low frequency sounds though as these are perceived through the bone, rather than through the air.

If your pet suffers from an aural hematoma (hemorrhage and bruising within the ear), then it may damage their ability to hear as this may lead to the breakage of blood vessels, blood clots, scarring and a thickened ear.

Just like in humans, the dog has three parts to their ear (also called an auricle). They are:

1. **External ear**

2. **Middle ear**

3. **Inner Ear**

1.   The External Ear

The external ear deals with the shape, size and mobility of the pet. It is the job of the outer ear to collect the sound waves and channel them to the middle ear (much like a big satellite dish). The ear is known as the *auricle,* or *pinna*, and it is an appendage on the side of the head. The auricle surrounds the external auditory canal. At the canal is the tympanic membrane, or *eardrum*. The eardrum acts as a barrier between the external (outer) ear and the middle ear.

Sound waves travel through the outer (external) ear and strike, or activate, the tympanic membrane. When the tympanic membrane is activated, it begins to vibrate.

The skin that lines the auditory canal has hair follicles, sebaceous glands (glands that produce sebum-an oily substance that lubricates hair and skin) and apocrine glands (sweat glands that become active during emotional stress and sexual stimulation). Pets that have more apocrine glands tend to have more ear problems than other breeds. One such breed is the spaniel.

The canine ear canal, just like those in humans, is designed to be self cleaning. If the canal suffers from chronic infections or inflammations, then it may lose its ability to self clean.

For breed standards, we look at the external ear as having position, shape and carriage.

- **Position**

- **Shape**

- **Carriage**

1. **Position**-the position of the ear is described as being **High** (joins the skull above the eyes as seen in Great Danes and Siberian Husky's); **Low** (joins skull below the eyes as seen in Basset Hounds and King Charles Spaniels); **Close** (ears are near the skull as seen in German Shepherds) and **Wide** (ears are far apart on the skull as seen in Italian Greyhounds)

2. **Shape**-there are a variety of ear shapes that include v-shaped, triangular, heart-shaped, tulip, rose and bat.

3. **Carriage**-ranges from 2" to 4 ½" and has a bend (or crook) in the middle. These descriptions include **Erect** (or pricked) like those of a German shepherd, **Dropped** like those of a Poodle and **Cocked** (semi-dropped/semi-pricked) like those of a Sheltie.

2. Middle Ear

The middle ear is a tiny epithelium lined cavity located in the hollow of the temporal bone. It contains four bones; the ossicles, malleus, incus and stapes. The oval window acts as a barrier between the middle ear and the inner ear.

As sound waves enters the ear it activates the tympanic membrane (eardrum) making it move back and forth slightly; the malleus takes the pressure from the tympanic membrane and passes it to the incus and then on to the stapes.

The stapes, or stirrups, are located at the end of the chain. The stapes vibrate at the same frequency as the eardrum, but approximately 20 times stronger. As the stapes strikes the oval window membrane, the membrane begins to vibrate. The pressure is then passed to the fluid within the cochlea.

The vibrations that are being transmitted have different frequencies, depending upon the sound that is received. Because of the length of the ear canal, the ear is capable of amplifying sounds frequencies.

3. The Inner Ear

The inner ear receives sounds and transforms the sound energy into internal vibrations of the bone structure of the middle ear. Here, sound energy is transformed into a compression wave, traveling like the coils of the Slinky (a coiled toy).

Within the inner ear the compression waves are then transformed within the inner ear fluid into nerve impulses, and then transmitted to the brain. The middle ear is a tiny epithelium lined cavity located in the hollow of the temporal bone. It contains four bones; the ossicles, malleus, incus and stapes. The oval window acts as a barrier between the middle ear and the inner ear.

The inner ear consists of three spaces called the bony labyrinth which is filled with a watery fluid called *perilymph*. The bony labyrinth is divided into three parts; the *vestibule*, *semicircular canals* and the *cochlea*. Within each of the canals is a specialized receptor called a *crista ampullaris*. The crista ampullaris generates nerve impulses when you move your head causing the sensory cells to become stimulated and the *endolymph* (thick fluid) to move.

The nerves from receptors in the vestibule join the nerves from the semicircular canals to form the vestibular nerve. The vestibular nerve joins with the cochlear nerve to form the cranial nerve VIII (otherwise referred to as the acoustic nerve). Nerve impulse passing through the cranial nerve VIII will eventually reach the cerebellum and medullar, while others will reach the cerebral cortex.

The organ of hearing is called the *organ of Corti*. The organ of Corti lies in the snail-shaped cochlea and is surrounded by endolymph. The organ of Corti contains more than 2,500 ciliated specialized sensory hair cells that create nerve impulses when they are contacted by the motion of sound waves.

So, as sound waves strike the tympanic membrane and cause it to vibrate, that vibration causes the oval window to vibrate. When the oval window vibrates, the perilymph in the bony labyrinth of the cochlea begins to move causing the endolymph in the cochlea to move. When the endolymph moves, sensory hair cells of the organ of Corti creates nerve impulses that travel over the cochlear nerve and become part of the *Cranial nerve VIII*. The Cranial nerve impulses are then translated into sound in the auditory cortex.

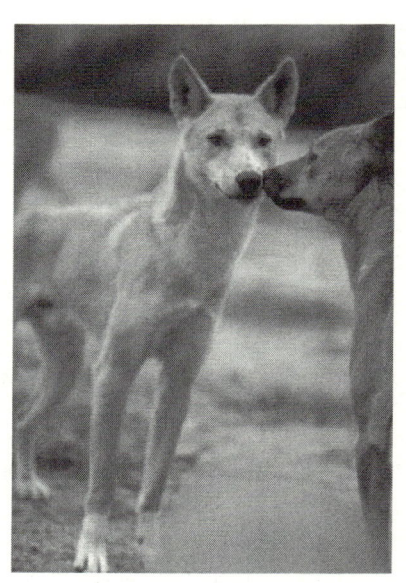

Chapter Four
The History of the Tuning Fork

According to the Wikipedia.org website on September 13, 2007, the definition it gives of the tuning fork is as follows:

*"A **tuning fork** is a simple metal two-pronged fork with the tines formed from a U-shaped bar of elastic material (usually steel). A tuning fork resonates at a specific constant pitch when set vibrating by striking it against a surface or with an object, and after waiting a moment to allow some high overtones to die out. The pitch that a particular tuning fork generates depends on the length of the two prongs, with two nodes near the bend of the U.*

When struck, it gives out a very faint note which is barely audible unless held close to the ear. For this reason, it is sometimes struck and then pressed down on a solid surface such as a desk which acts as a sounding board and greatly amplifies the note."

Tuning forks are used to tune musical instruments and are also used in physics classrooms across the country to teach students about sound, vibration and sound waves.

In the medical field, tuning forks such as the C-512 Hz were used by health care practitioners to make assertations of a patient's hearing. While the higher tuning fork frequencies checked for hearing loss, other lower sounding tuning forks, such as the C-128 Hz, were used to check vibration sense generally as part of the examination of the peripheral nervous system. In some parts of the world, tuning forks have since been replaced by machinery to perform these same tasks.

The tuning fork was first invented in 1711 in England by Royal Sergeant Trumpeter to the court and luteist, John Shore. At the time, he jokingly called it a pitch fork. It was made of steel and had a pitch of A423.5.

But the thoughts and beliefs about tuning forks can be traced much further back in time; All the way back in fact to the early Greeks. In 583 B.C., the Greek philosopher, Pythagoras, made a device called the monochord and set the pitch to 256 Hz. The Greek and Egyptians used the monochord to make intricate mathematical calculations.

But other uses for sound and vibrations began to surface. In 1550 Pacia, Italy, the physician, mathematician and astrologer Girolamo Cardano, noticed how sound was being perceived through the skin.

Just three years later, in 1553 Paua, Italy, H. Capivacci, a physician noticed that this knowledge of sound that was being perceived through the skin might be used as a diagnostic tool for differentiating between hearing disorders located in the middle ear or in the acoustic nerve. (Many people living today can remember having their hearing tested by a doctor holding a tuning fork.)

In the 18th century the German physicist Ernest Chladni, discovered that when a violin bow was drawn vertically across the rim of a metal plate, the sound waves it produced created patterns in the sand that was sprinkled on the plate. For each different musical tone that was played, the sand particles formed a different geometric pattern.

In the late 1960s, the Swiss scientist Hans Jenny discovered that the low frequency sounds produced simple geometric shapes and as the sound frequency increased, the shapes become more complex. He also found that the sound 'OH' produced a perfect circle and that the sound 'OM' produced a pattern similar to that of the ancient Indian mandala for 'OM.'

In 1974, a professional jazz musician named Fabien Maman noticed that by playing certain musical notes he could have an energizing effect on the audience.

In the late 1970s, Fabien joined with the senior researcher at the National Centre for Scientific Research in Paris, Helene Grimal, to study the effects of sound on normal and malignant cells.

The pair used all types of sound making instruments including flutes, drums, gongs and more. They discovered that at 30-40 decibels, the sound always produced changes in the cells and that the higher up the musical scale they went, the frequency would travel outward from the center of the cell to its outer membrane. The most amazing results happened when the human voice was used.

In an experiment on female volunteers with breast cancer, women were taught to tone the whole scale using a violin to keep a base note for 21 minutes at a time. They spent 3 ½ hours a day for one month toning. One woman's tumor disappeared completely. (4)

On the cellular level, Fabien Maman found that the note 'C' made the cells longer, that the note 'D' produced a variety of colors in the cells; the 'A' note changed the color of the cell's energy field from red to pink, and that the note 'E' made the cells spherical. Maman also noticed that the note 'F' made the cells round, balanced and with vibrant colors of magenta and turquoise. He also noted that the 'F' note was the fundamental sound of the singer and believed that this was helpful for the physical body through its harmonizing and regenerating effect at the cellular level. (5)

The Japanese scientist, Masaru Emoto, discovered that music affected water and that different types of music affected it in different ways. While he found that classical music, folk music and mantras produced beautiful crystals and colors; heavy metal music produced patterns that appeared exploded and shattered.

With our bodies made up of more than 60% water, Emoto's work demonstrated the importance of how our body is influenced by the sounds around us and by the information stored in the water that we drink.

In his book, *The Mozart Effect*, Don Campbell showed how music has beneficial effects for human health. From improving concentration to enhancing our intuition, music can affect our bodies.

Slow tempo music slows the heart rate and breathing patterns. It calms our nervous systems and even affects our metabolism. Music can also effect our emotions. Campbell found that by playing music in the dentist's office or operating room, patients were better able to remain calm.

Dr. Tomatis used high frequency sounds (3,000 Hz. and above) to activate the brain and affect cognitive functions such as thinking, spatial perception and memory. Listening to these sounds increases our attentiveness and concentration. (2)

Barbara Hero and the International Lambdoma Research Institute in Kennebunk, Maine, discovered that by passing sound waves through each organ of the body that they were able to calculate the optimal frequency for each of the organs using mathematical formulas based on the speed of sound.

Chapter Five
The Tuning Fork

Parts of the Tuning Fork

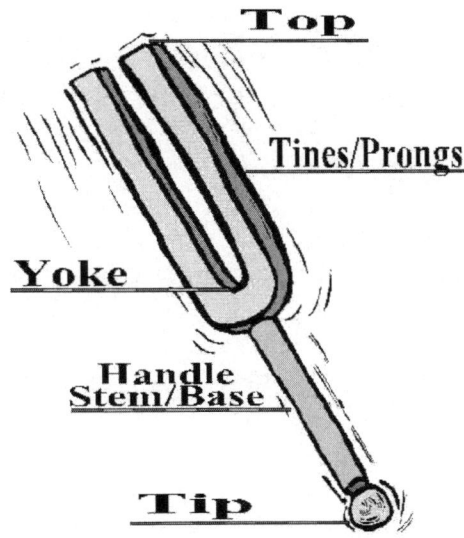

Take your tuning fork in your hand and look at the different parts of the instrument. The very top of the tuning fork is called the *top*. The two long sides of the tuning fork are called *prongs* or *tines*. They are responsible for creating the vibrations of your tuning fork.

Follow these two prongs down you will come to a U-shaped part of the tuning fork that we call the *yoke*. The bottom part of the tuning fork is called the *stem*, or *handle.* This is where you hold your tuning fork to activate it. The very end of the handle is sometimes called the *'Tip'* of the tuning fork. So when I say to place the tip of the tuning fork on the body, this is the part that you will be using.

Calibrating Tuning Forks

A tuning fork should provide a stable pitch reference with absolute accuracy when it is properly cared for.

What kinds of thing affect the pitch of a tuning fork?

The largest effect on tuning forks is the temperature. The pitch of the tuning fork can drop one percent for every eight-degree rise in temperature Fahrenheit. This can occur most easily in the northern states where you may take your tuning forks from your climate-controlled home, into your cold car, from the now warm car and through the cold air, back into another climate-controlled area (or forget about them and leave them in the cold car). These things happen, and you should know that they will affect the pitch of your tuning forks.

Is there anything I can do to fix the pitch of my tuning fork?

Yes.

If the pitch of your fork needs to be lowered, then you will want to put a notch between the two tines. If you want to raise the pitch of your fork, then you will want to file or grind some metal from the top ends of the fork to make them shorter. The shorter the tuning forks, the higher the pitch.

If you file or grind some of the metal from one tine, try to remove exactly the same amount of metal from the other tine. This will keep your fork balanced. If you notch one side of the fork, it is a good idea to notch the other side as well to maintain symmetry.

Proper Storage of your Tuning Forks

Store your tuning forks in a clean and dry place. Pitch varies with temperature, so try to keep your tuning forks stored at the same moderate temperature. Condensation due to cold may cause discoloration and corrosion. Excessive force should not be used when toning.

Always use a rubber mallet, the palm of your hand, a tuning fork activator, the front muscle on the top of your leg, a rubber hockey puck, or even the rubber heel of a boot as a striking place for your tuning forks. DO NOT clean your tuning forces with detergent, ammonia, or other chemicals

You can store your tuning forks in the wooden box or in the canvas wrap-around they came in. I store one set of my tuning forks in an upright position in a block of wood into which holes have been drilled.

I purchased this block of wood on-line, but if you are creative enough, you can make your own by drilling holes into a simple scrap piece of wood. I have found this to be handy for times when I need to hear a quick tone.

Precautions

Until further studies are done in using tuning forks, I would **NOT** use Tuning Forks on the following groups of people: Those with pacemakers, metal implants, metal pins or other metal bindings, and pregnant women.

Please note that is my own feeling on the subject, which may or may not be found to be true. I have always believed that if you should err; err on the side of caution.

How to Hold your Tuning Forks

The Correct Way to Hold your Tuning Fork

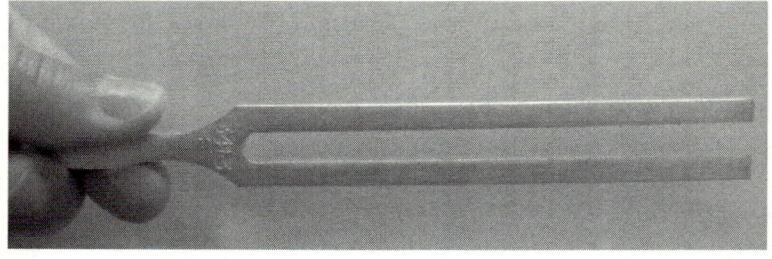

Do Hold Fork at End of Handle. Keep wrist loose.

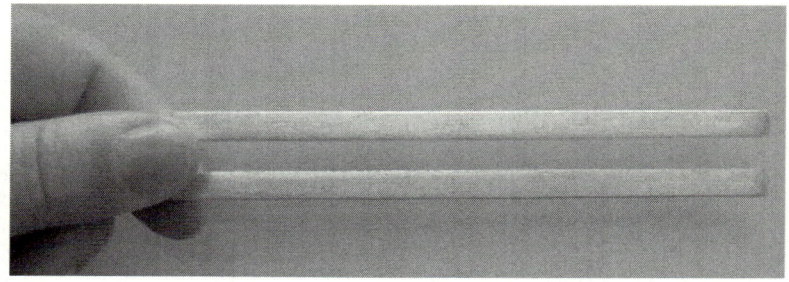

Do <u>not</u> grab the tuning fork up close to the tines.

It may take some time to feel comfortable holding and activating your tuning forks. Do not become discouraged. With practice you will become confident in using them. You may wish to try using the unweighted tuning forks first before moving on to the weighted tuning forks. Unweighted tuning forks are much lighter and easier to hold for long periods of time.

Instructions for Toning the Tuning Fork

1. Use the Tuning Fork Activator

2. Use a Rubber Mallet

3. Tap the fork on your leg muscle

4. Tap the fork on the palm of your hand

5. Gently tap two (or more) forks together.

(Please note that tapping two forks together may cause them to chip or dent, and then they will lose their pitch and tone.)

PLEASE remember-Do **NOT** activate tuning forks near your pet's ear. The sound may cause irritation or discomfort to your pet.

How to Activate your Tuning Fork

The surface you choose to activate your tuning fork with is very important. The harder the surface you use to activate your tuning fork, the louder, crisper and longer the tone/vibrations will be. The softer the surface you choose to activate your tuning fork, the softer, muted and shorter the tone/vibrations will be.

Since you are doing healing sessions for the client's enjoyment and healing and NOT your own, you will find that there will be times when a client can become easily agitated with specific sounds. In these cases, it would benefit the client to have these specific notes muted and softened (or not used at all until another session.)

In the same way, you will find that you will need to amplify the note/vibration of the tuning fork that you are using for the client. If this happens, then you will look for a harder surface in which to activate your tuning fork.

In addition to the surface that you choose to activate your tuning fork, the place along the tines that you strike the activator with will also affect the quality, crispness and loudness of your tone/vibrations.

The further up the tines that you go to strike your tuning fork, the less crisp and softer the tone/vibrations will become. The lower you go down the tines to the yoke, the more muted and less vibrations you will receive.

The actual perfect place to strike your tuning fork is approximately 1/3 the distance up from the yoke (or 2/3 down from the top of the tine). Practice will make perfect so go ahead and explore this wonderful area of sound therapy.

NOTE: Please do **NOT** activate your tuning fork on your knee cap.

Hard Surfaces

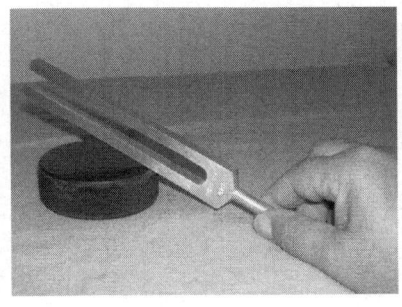 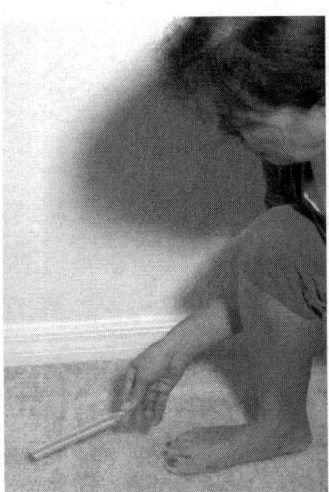

#1   #2

A common hockey puck or a carpeted floor makes a great activator for the tuning fork. Even though the hockey puck it is what I consider a 'hard' surface, it's rubber material makes for a softer sounding 'loud' sound than the floor does. Even a block of wood can be used as an activator for the tuning fork. Considered a 'hard' surface, the block of wood has natural cushioning that allows for a softer sound.

To Activate:

In the #1 picture you can see that the tuning fork is being activated two-thirds of the way down from the top. This is the ideal method of activating a tuning fork of this type. As you go through the other manuals, you will be instructed on how to activate other types of tuning forks that will be more popular due to their style.

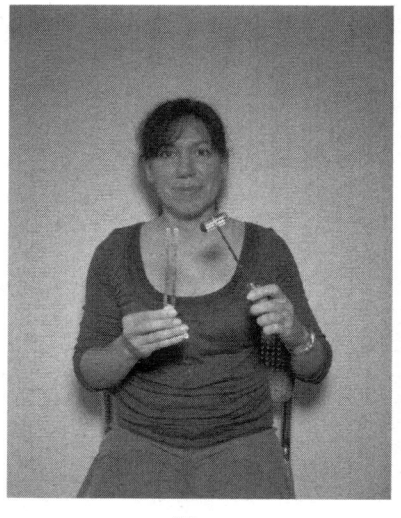 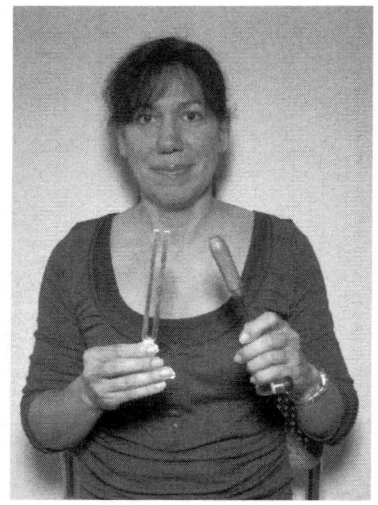

#2   #3

#1. For those of you who have a wooden mallet with a rubber tip on one side, you can activate your tuning fork by holding the fork in one hand and 'striking' the fork with the rubber end of the mallet in your other hand.

#2. As another option, turn your mallet around and strike the tuning fork with the wooden handle of your mallet.

Notes: Can you see or hear a difference when you strike the tuning fork with the rubber or wooden side of the mallet?

As you work with your tuning forks in actual client sessions, you will notice that there are times when you need to activate your tuning forks using a hard surface while there will be times to use a softer surface.

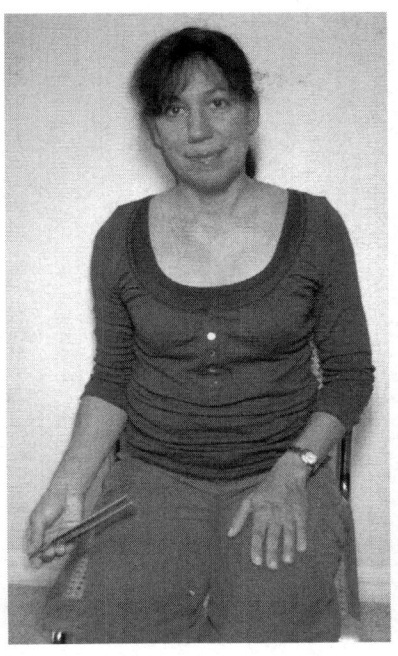 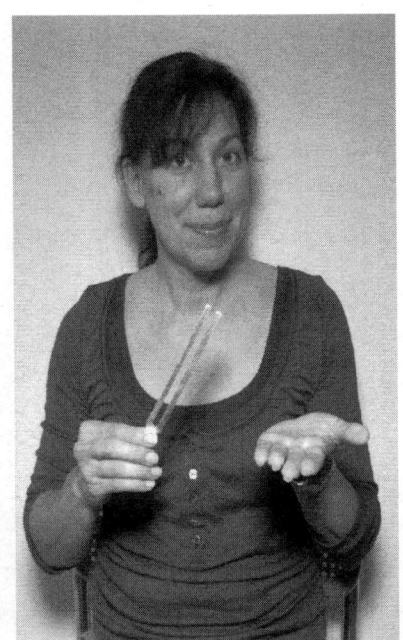

#4   **#5**

You can also use the top of your thigh or the meaty palm of your hand. This is a very 'soft' surface and the sound and vibrations from your tuning fork will be very soft and muted.

When you have a client who is very ill, a muted sound is often the most healing sound to them. I have seen other practitioners using loud clanging sounds and have seen their clients grimace under the sounds. Believe me; they won't come back for more of that.

The sounds coming from the tuning fork will be very soft and muted. When deciding on which activator to use, keep the client's needs in mind-not your own need to 'hear' loud tones.

Ways to Use your Tuning Forks

1. Place the handle of a vibrating tuning fork on a specific chakra.

2. Place the handle of vibrating tuning fork on reflex points.

3. Place the handle of a vibrating tuning fork on a muscle.

4. Place the handle of vibrating tuning fork on acupuncture points

5. Use a vibrating tuning fork on bodies of water.

6. Place the handle of a vibrating tuning fork on a bone.

7. Wave a vibrating tuning fork over a specific area of the body.

8. Wave a vibrating tuning fork over the auric layers of the body.

9. Wave a vibrating tuning fork over water before you drink it.

10. Wave a vibrating tuning fork over your food before you eat it.

11. Use two or more vibrating tuning forks on the meridian system of the body.

12. Use a vibrating tuning fork with a crystal to direct healing.

13. Use a vibrating tuning fork to remove negative and stagnant energy in a room.

14. Use a vibrating tuning fork to clear and energize crystals and gemstones.

15. Use a vibrating tuning fork to prepare for a meditation session

16. Use a vibrating tuning fork on reflex points on the feet.

17. Use a vibrating tuning fork on reflex points on the hands.

18. Use a vibrating tuning fork on the chakras

19. Use a vibrating tuning fork on pets and wildlife.

20. Use a vibrating tuning fork on plants.

Chapter Six

Elements and Tuning Fork Association

Elements and Tuning Fork Association

Every tuning fork is associated with one of the specific elements. The elements are: Earth, Water, Fire, Air, and Ether. Synergies are the mutually reinforcing action of separate substances that, together, produce an effect greater than that of all the components (or parts) acting separately.

By combining two tuning forks and playing them together, you are creating a synergy. Synergies are also popular in numerous alternative therapies, such as Aromatherapy and Bach Flower Remedies.

Through combining certain sounds, one can achieve specific results in a shorter period of time. Using two forks at the same time is not always preferred over using a single fork. You will have to judge for yourself and for your client which is in the best interest for the healing session.

Please keep in mind that not all people enjoy sound therapy sessions. For some people, specific tones and overtones can cause them distress in the session. If you combine more than one fork at a time, you will also double the chances that your client will not benefit from the healing session at all due to physical discomfort. You will have to intuit what is the right thing to do for your client.

It is for this reason that I use the beginner/basic set of tuning forks. These tuning forks are the lightest in weight and they create the softest of sounds. If a client is comfortable with this set of tuning forks, then I can use the heavier and louder tuning forks. Remember, these healing sessions are for the client's highest good, not yours. Please keep your client's overall well being and comfort in mind when creating a healing session. Not everyone enjoys long-clanging tuning forks!

Single Forks and their Elemental Associations

The "C" Tuning Fork (Middle/Low)-256 Hz.

Element is Fire

Associated with the Sacral Plexus

Associated with the Adrenal Gland

Affects the Elimination System of the Body

Affects the Lymph and Skeletal System of the Body

Associated with the Sense of Smell

Affects the Physical Body in the Auric Field

Color is Red

Use this Tuning Fork to:

Burn out Cancer in the body

Warm Cold areas of the body

> Foot, leg, knee and ankle problems

> Adrenal problems

> Weight issues (obesity)

Poor circulation

Paranoia & Neurosis

Eating disorders

Hemorrhoids, Diarrhea & Constipation

Sciatica

The "D" Tuning Fork - 288 Hz.

Element is Water

Associated with the Lumbar Plexus

Associated with the Gonads

Affects the Reproductive System

Affects the Assimilation of Food in the Body

Associated with the Sense of Taste

Affects the Etheric Body of the Auric Field

Color is Orange

Use this Tuning Fork to:

Increase overall immunity

Eating disorders

Impotency, Infertility, Reproductive problems

Kidney problems, Bladder problems

Diabetes

Muscular system problems

Sexual problems

Frigidity

The "E" Tuning Fork - 320 Hz.

Element is Fire
Associated with the Solar Plexus
Associated with the Pancreas
Affects the Muscular System
Affects the Digestive System
Associated with the Sense of Sight
Affects the Emotional Body of the Auric Field
Color is Yellow

Use this Tuning Fork to:

Pancreas

Adrenals, Spleen

Gall Bladder

Skin problems, Small Intestine

Hypoglycemia

Stomach, Liver

Diabetes

Ulcers

Nerves

The "F" Tuning Fork - 341-3 Hz

Element is Air
Associated with the Cardiac Plexus
Associated with the Thymus
Affects the Nervous System
Affects the Circulation System
Affects the Immune System
Associated with the Sense of Touch
Affects the Mental Body of the Auric Field
Color is Green

Use this Tuning Fork to:
Thymus, Glands
Heart & Cardiac Plexus, Stroke, Blood pressure
Asthma, Pneumonia, Bronchitis. Allergies, Lungs,
Respiratory problems
Emotional disorders
Arthritis
Relationship problems

The "G" Tuning Fork - 384 Hz.

Element is Air

Associated with the Cervical Plexus

Affects the Growth and Metabolism System of the Body

Associated with the Thyroid

Associated with the Sense of Hearing

Affects the Astral Body of the Auric Field

Color is Blue

Use this Tuning Fork to:

Calm an agitated area in the body

Cool an inflamed area in the body

Fevers in the body

Throat, Vocal chords, Esophagus, Laryngitis, Sore throat

Voice problems

Mouth problems, Teeth problems

Thyroid, Parathyroid

Asthma, Allergies

Flu

Vertigo

Anemia

The "A" Tuning Fork - 426-6 Hz.

Element is Fire

Associated with the Carotid Plexus

Associated with the Pituitary Gland

Affects the Endocrine System

Associated with the Sense of Sight

Affects the Etheric Template Body of the Auric Field

Color is Indigo

Use this Tuning Fork to:

Congested head

Sinus problems

Headaches

Ear problems and diseases

Eye problems and diseases

Nose problems and diseases

Insomnia

Mental problems

Skeletal system

Pituitary gland, Pineal gland

The "B" Tuning Fork - 480 Hz.

Element is Water
Associated with the Brain
Associated with the Pineal Gland
Affects the Nervous System of the Body
Associated with the Sense of Feeling
Affects the Celestial Body of the Auric Field
Color is Violet

Use this Tuning Fork to:

Nervous problems
Depression, Insanity, Psychosis
Worry
Insomnia
Brain tumors
Cerebral tumors
Cranial pressure
Epilepsy
Pain
Rheumatism
Pineal gland

NOTES:

Chapter Seven

What is Acupuncture?

History of Acupuncture (on animals)

Acupuncture, the healing art of inserting needles into specific points on the body, dates back to ancient China. The word Acupuncture comes from the Latin word, *acus*, meaning "needle" and *pungere*, which means "prick."

In China, the use of acupuncture is intended to help the body use its own innate ability to bring health and well-being to areas in need. The practice of using needles on points of the body dates back before the Han Dynasty (202 B.C.). But it is Shun Yang (480 BC) from China who is considered by many to be the father of veterinary acupuncture. The oldest known text book is the 'Huang-Ti Nei-Jeng Tsu-Wen,' which outlined the theory and practice of acupuncture for humans in a question and answer format.

From China, acupuncture knowledge spread to India where the earliest records of veterinary acupuncture was recorded for the treatment of elephants, some 3000 years ago.

From Asia, acupuncture spread to the West (North America) where Sir William Osler, an instructor at both Harvard and Yale University, wrote on the subject of acupuncture in 1836. It wasn't until 1926 that his writings made it into the New England Journal of Medicine.

Even thought the American Medical Association Council of Scientific Affairs declared acupuncture to be an experimental medical procedure in 1973, it was the American Osteopathic Association who endorsed the use of acupuncture in 1983 as part of a medical practice.

In ancient China, acupuncturist once used spikes of fishbone to perform acupuncture. These bones were used and reused for many years. Today, trained acupuncturists use disposable (single-use) needles usually made from stainless steel that has an approximate diameter of .01" to .02". For very fine needles, a thicker wire is attached to the very top of the needle to allow for strength and durability at a place where the therapist needs to hold on to it. Sometimes this wire is made from bronze.

The Chinese term zhēn jǐu (針灸), which was commonly used to refer to acupuncture, comes from the word *zhen* meaning "needle," and the word *jiu* which means "moxibustion".

In traditional Chinese medicine, the needles were warmed before use. One way of warming the needles was by a process called **moxibustion** (burning of mugwort).

One method of using moxibustion was to tie the dried herb (mugwort) to the end of the acupuncture needle, insert the needle into the body, and ignite the mugwort. After the mugwort was producing a good flame, you would then blow the flame out and allow the mugwort to smolder for a few minutes.

The heat created by the smoldering moxibustion would warm the tissue that surrounded the inserted needle. Even though this is a great tool to use for humans, it is not one that I would recommend using for pets. In addition to the primal fear of fire and smoke, the use of moxibustion on animals may lead to unintentional burning of the animals' fur. If you do choose to use moxibustion on your animals, please be sure to watch them carefully and have a pail of water, or fire extinguisher handy in case the animal bolts away from you.

Even though the practice of acupuncture began on humans; it was later used on animals. In China, acupuncture was used on horses and other farm animals before being adopted for use on dogs, cats, ferrets, birds, etc.

Based on the concept of Qi (universal life force energy), acupuncture was believed to open stagnate or blocked areas of energy in the body in order to release Qi.

The word Qi is pronounced '*chee*.' The release of Qi in the body would then help boost the body's immune system, release endorphins and hormones, increase circulation, and more.

But the release of Qi doesn't just increase the flow of energy; it can also balance, tone and sedate it. Using acupuncture, you can decrease inflammation, lower high blood pressure, and bring tone and balance to organs.

Qi travels through the body in pathways called **meridians**. In study, there are 12 major meridians in the human body. The Chinese have long understood about the meridians as energy pathways in the body and have used this knowledge to help in the healing process of humans.

It was discovered that animals also have very similar meridians through which Qi flows. Because of this, it was understood that acupuncture can also be used on animals to activate, stimulate, tone, balance and sedate specific points along the meridians.

When we talk about specific points, we are referring to reflex-points, or points that are traditionally called "acupuncture points" in English, or "xue" (穴, cavities) in Chinese.

There are more than 365 points in the human (and animal) body. Each of these points has a Chinese name, a translated name, and an organ point number. One example is the point known as Wind Pond, or otherwise referred to as GB20. These points lie beneath the skin and are connected to organs, muscles, joints and the nervous system.

Thanks in part to the work of Austrian born acupuncturist Oswald Kothbauer and German acupuncturist Erwin Westermayer, the treatment of cattle and horses using acupuncture became recognized as an alternative modality. Through their work, a more modern day acceptance of animal acupuncture was born.

Acupuncture for Animal

Using acupuncture needles on animals become widely accepted in the U.S. some thirty years ago. In 1974, the International Veterinary Acupuncture Society (IVAS), a non-profit organization dedicated to promoting excellence in the practice of veterinary acupuncture, was formed. To date, the IVAS is the only international veterinary acupuncture organization of its kind with more than 150,000 vets and 700,000 par veterinary assistants in several different countries.

The IVAS establishes standards practice for its membership offering educational programs and accreditation examination. According to its website, www.ivas.org, the Society seeks to integrate veterinary acupuncture and the practice of western veterinary science. Although the use of acupuncture is indicated for mostly functional problems such as allergies, pain, inflammation and paralysis, the Society further lists conditions for which acupuncture is indicated. These conditions include:

- Musculoskeletal problems, such as arthritis

- vertebral disc pathology, Sore backs

- Skin problems, such as lick granuloma

- Respiratory problems, such as feline asthma

- Gastrointestinal problems, such as diarrhea

- Selected reproductive problems and disorders

- Nervous system problems, such as facial nerve paralysis

- Allergic dermatitis

- Heaves

- "Bleeders"

- Gastrointestinal problems, such as nonsurgical colic

Acupuncture can stimulate nerves, increase blood circulation, relieve muscle spasm, and cause the release of hormones, such as endorphins (one of the body's pain control chemicals) and cortisol (a natural steroid).

Using tuning forks on animals, instead of needles, will accomplish much the same effect but without pain or risks. Since tuning forks are NOT an invasive procedure, there are many risks that you will not have to worry about.

Some risks of using needles include creating a hematoma if you accidentally puncture a circulatory structure, brain damage or stroke from deep needling at the base of the skull, nerve injury from accidental puncture of a nerve, kidney damage from deep needling of the lower back, pneumothorax from deep needling into the lung, etc.

In addition to the physical trauma of improper needling, there is also a hygienic concern to using needles. Without proper sterilization procedures, needles may transfer diseases such as the HIV virus and hepatitis. There are stringent codes of safe practice for practitioner to follow in the use of needles in acupuncture treatment. But when using tuning forks, the codes are a lot less stringent. For proper cleaning of tuning forks, I suggest to wipe your tuning forks before and after every treatment session with an alcohol wipe.

Acupuncture may be one of the safest and effective forms of treatment for animals when administered properly. Using the basis knowledge of acupuncture, you can substitute needles for tuning forks making the outcome even more profound. Adding tuning forks adds an additional layer of sound and vibration to the healing session.

What to Look for in a Session

Should an animal become lethargic or sleepy after a session, it is an indication of a physiological change happening. These animals may present with lethargy for approximately 24 hours after a treatment session but this will often pass in time.

Length of Frequency of Treatment Session

How long you should keep using tuning forks on your pet, and how often you should give them a treatment, depends upon the condition that you are treating. Stimulation of a single acupuncture point may take anywhere from 10 seconds to 20 minutes or more. A simple ache, sprain, or pain point may require only one treatment session while other more serious or chronic conditions may require several treatment sessions.

When several treatment sessions are called for, the first several treatments are usually longer in duration and are done with greater frequency (such as 1-3 sessions per week for 4 weeks). After a positive outcome is witnessed, treatment sessions may then be tapered down to 1 session per month, ending with 1 session per 6 months. Positive results should be seen by the third treatments session.

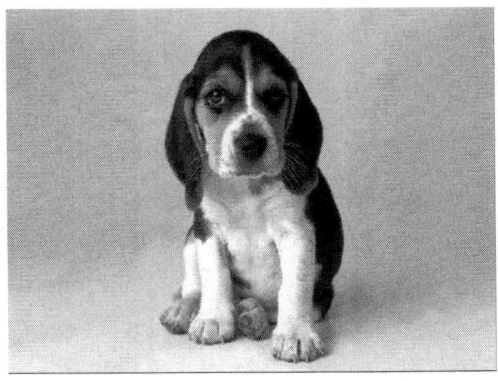

Chronic and Acute Conditions

Acupuncture has been found effective in treating a variety of chronic and even acute conditions. Acute conditions are those that arise suddenly and are intense for a short period of time. Chronic conditions are those that happen over a long period of time. This will also hold true for using tuning forks to treat these conditions. Some chronic and acute conditions that acupuncture and tuning forks can help include:

- Orthopedic, obstetric, and surgical pain

- Paralysis

- Noninfectious inflammation

- Allergies

- Arthritis

- Disc problems

- Gastrointestinal problems, such as <u>vomiting</u> and <u>diarrhea</u>

- Male and female reproductive problems

- Skin disease

- Incontinence

- Hearing loss

- Cardiovascular disorders

- Chronic respiratory conditions, such as asthma

- Musculoskeletal disorders

- Neurological disorders

Chapter Eight

Acupuncture/Sound Session

The work of the acupuncture/sound therapist is to restore the energy flow, balance and rhythm to the body. In this way, the body will be able to carry out its many healing processes. But acupuncture and sound therapy are NOT stand alone modalities. All modalities work in tandem with diet, exercise, proper environment, etc. This course is truly a 'holistic' practice.

The practice of acupuncture has grown significantly in mainstream practice. For many individuals who are considering becoming a veterinary, they may find a chapter or two of their textbooks devoted to the practice and wisdom of acupuncture. One latest survey predicted that approximately 3 million veterinarians, assistants, and medical practitioners worldwide practice acupuncture.

In practicing Acupuncture, therapists first determine the cause of any imbalances in the Qi, life force energy. This determination is called the **etiology** of the disease. It is extremely helpful to the practitioner to find the cause of any discomfort or ailment in order to properly treat it. I often tell my own students to search out the 'root' cause of the illness in order to successfully remove it from the individual, or animal. Sometimes locating this root cause may take more time than you would think. It involves looking at the client, listening to the client, hearing the client, smelling the client, etc. There are many 'clues' that you would look for before you would make a final conclusion as to the treatment plan.

A typical visit to a 'holistic' veterinarian's office may include the following:

- Animal is placed on examining table where its temperature is taken, a physical exam is performed, heart is listened to, bowel sounds are listened to, and the abdomen is palpated to check for any masses. Lab test may be ordered.

- The practitioner would then ask about the dog's behavior and previous history. Asks about the dogs' sleeping patterns, surface preferences to lie on, diet, the animals' environment, stressors, checking tongue, looking at animals body shape, skin and coat. Taking a look at the overall presence of the animal (jittery, lethargic, etc.). Checks the dog's pulse and points along the back that correspond to specific internal organs.

- Check for odors from eyes, nose, ears and mouth.

A typical visit to an acupuncture/tuning fork practitioner would include:

•   Animal is placed on examining table where its temperature is taken, a physical exam is performed, heart is listened to, bowel sounds are listened to, and the abdomen is palpated to check for any masses. Lab test may be ordered.

•   The practitioner would then ask about the dog's behavior and previous history. Asks about the dogs' sleeping patterns, surface preferences to lie on, diet, the animals' environment, stressors, checking tongue, looking at animals body shape, skin and coat. Taking a look at the overall presence of the animal (jittery, lethargic, etc.). Checks the dog's pulse and points along the back that correspond to specific internal organs.

•   Check for odors from eyes, nose, ears and mouth.

•   Decision on which tuning forks to use on which point on the body, the length and frequency of the sound therapy session.

An example of the difference between Traditional Chinese Medicine (TCM) and Western Medicine would be the following: An animal presents with frequent urination. The Western Medicine would treat with medicine based upon the size of the animal. In TCM, the frequent urination is viewed as a weakness in the kidney yang causing an overall deficiency in the animals' Qi.

Depending upon the size and location of the points to be treated, different needle lengths are chosen. The animal would then return for follow up sessions of 15 seconds to 30 minutes, with more frequent visits in the beginning and then bringing the visits down to twice a year, until the goal was achieved and maintained.

In 1980, a study was written by The University of California (UCLA), in Los Angeles. The study was conducted by the UCLA Acupuncture Research Project (1973-1980) to determine what, if any, help can be achieved using acupuncture on clients. It was discovered that acupuncture helped in the treatment of chronic pain, hearing loss, bronchial asthma and in compulsive disorders such as drug and tobacco addiction and obesity.

Additional studies showed acupuncture to be beneficial for humans and animals alike in the treatment of pain and inflammatory conditions. For these conditions, acupuncture acted as an analgesic for pain and as an anti-inflammatory medication. This held true in treating arthritic conditions in both human and animals.

Conditions for non-treatment of animals

There are some conditions to which using acupuncture philosophy and tuning forks would not be appropriate for some animals. These situations include times when the animal is in an extremely volatile or excitable condition that they are secreting their own adrenaline (which would counteract what you are trying to achieve).

Other conditions would include if the animal was already taking certain medications such as corticosteroids, which would decrease the pain sensor receptors. Pain among animals depends upon the kind of breeds you are working, as well as, their sex. Female animals have a much higher pain threshold than their male counterparts.

Acupuncture and the Athlete

Acupuncture may be used to improve the performances of animals, especially for racing horses and dogs. For those who choose to use acupuncture, or in the case of this course, tuning forks to improve the performance of racers, it is suggested to treat the animal at least 2-3 days BEFORE the event and NOT directly before the event itself.

The reason it is suggested to NOT use tuning forks before an important event is that tuning forks, just like acupuncture, can have a very sedating effect on the body. But after the sedating and/or balancing phase is over, there is an increase in circulation and vitality with an overall feeling of energy and well-being. This is the best way to feel for an important race or competition.

For animals that are undergoing training, it can be beneficial to give the animal acupuncture treatment sessions twice a week to once a month. This would depend upon the intensity and duration of the training.

Regular acupuncture treatment sessions can help the animal by treating any minor injuries as they occur. These treatment sessions would help to keep muscles and tendons resistant to injury. Keeping your animals in tip top physical condition will help them compete in athletic competition or in showing contests.

How an acupuncture/tuning fork session works

When you take your animal for an acupuncture/Tuning Fork Therapy® session, your animal should have a complete history taken. The therapist should look at your pet for external signs of illness. These external signs include the color of the animal's coat (dull), eyes, breathing patterns, and discharges from eyes, nose or mouth.

The therapist should also ask you about your animal's medical history, its daily routines and schedules, diet, and overall behavior. After reviewing their notes and asking any additional questions, a course of action should be written up as a plan for the animal.

The first session will of course be longer in duration than any future sessions would be since the therapists needs to do all of their preliminary work on the animal's first visit.

The Tuning Fork Session itself should only last for up to 20 minutes. If a longer session is called for, then of course the practitioner can continue, but few animals will remain willing participants for longer than 20 minutes.

Most animals will leave the session as soon as they have received enough energy for their body at the time. No matter how short the session may appear to you-know that the benefits from the session will continue for another 12-24 hours after the first session, and longer for future ones.

Be realistic in your expectations of positive results. It is very rare for an animal to be 100% cured from any ailment, issue or problem in the first session. Since no two animals are exactly the same, there is just no way to calculate how many sessions any one animal will need to have to overcome their condition.

Positive results should be seen at least by the third treatment session. If your animal is not showing signs of improvement after the third treatment session, then you should revisit the history of the animal and reevaluate your first findings. Perhaps there is another way to treat the animal such as using a different frequency fork over a different acupuncture point.

After an animal has presented with a positive outcome, it would still be wise to have the animal still receive a treatment session at least twice a year to maintain the positive outcome. Please note that in cases of chronic disease, such as arthritis, it may take weeks to see any positive changes occur in the animal.

For animals, using tuning forks on acupuncture points may help the following conditions:

- arthritis, osteoarthritis
- muscular injuries
- reproductive issues, infertility, male impotence and libido
- hormonal issues, normalize blood sugar levels
- thyroid, pituitary and parathyroid functions
- immunity and adrenal functions
- behavior disorders
- insomnia
- skin conditions
- digestive disorders
- urinary problems, elimination problems
- respiratory issues, asthma, allergies, Sinusitis
- fatigue and vitality issues
- performance issues

- traveling problems
- heart conditions, canine stroke
- back problems, spinal problems
- Canine Epilepsy, CDRM, Chorea, CMO
- Craniomandibular Osteopathy
- Cruciate Ligament
- Degenerative Disc and Joint Disease
- Disc Disease
- Prolapse
- DJD
- Dry Eye, Eye issues
- Glaucoma
- Elbow Dysplasia, Hip Dysplasia, Fibrous Dysplasia
- Enuresis
- Eosinophilic Myositis
- Epilepsy
- Horners Syndrome
- Incontinence
- IVDD
- KCS
- Keratoconjunctivitis Sicca
- Laryngeal Paralysis
- Ligament Injury
- Meningitis
- Myositis
- Non-Union Fracture
- OCD
- Osteochondritis Dissecans
- Osteodystrophy
- Paralysis
- Shaker Syndrome
- Spondylitis
- Spondylosis
- Spondylopathy
- Sprain

- Syringomyelia
- Ununited anconeal process
- Vestibular Syndrome
- Wobbler Syndrome

Chapter Nine

10 Acupuncture points for Sound Healing

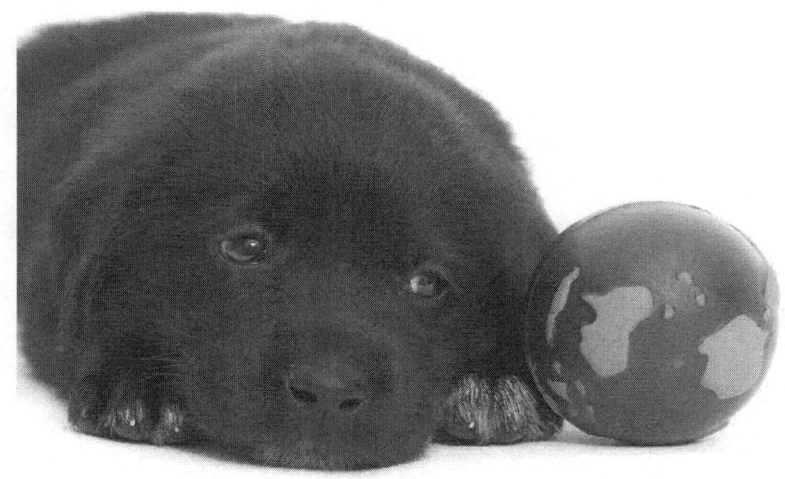

Animal Acupuncture is a holistic, or 'wholistic,' view of treating the entire animal. Where emotions are involved, you add additional alternative modalities such as Reiki or Bach Flower remedies.

When we view the animal and their specific needs in a holistic way, we are not just isolating the symptom, behavior, or disease. We are looking for a whole range of signs, events and temperament in making a final decision as to how to proceed in the treatment of the animal.

If you are familiar with the use of acupuncture modalities (which is out of the scope of this specific course) then you can use the Five Element theory, Yin or Yang, Excess or Deficient, Hot or Cold, Windy or Damp, Internal or External, etc.

For those who are not so familiar with acupuncture, that is alright as this course deals with the use of tuning forks on specific points on an animal rather than the entire acupressure philosophy of diagnosing the problem.

If you are familiar with acupuncture, then you can use your current knowledge to help you in selecting the correct tuning fork for the outcome that you wish to achieve.

Yin is passive, cold (low body temperature) and calm. Yan is like fire and it is hot (fever or inflammation, aggression), active and excitable. Deficient conditions are said to be Yin and include lethargy, lack of get up and go, weak bark or meow, general weakness, etc.

Overactive conditions are said to be Yang and include a full strong bark or meow, hyperactivity, aggressiveness, etc. Yin is related to internal functions of the body that are chronic (lasting longer than one month) such as diabetes. Yang affects the outside of the body and is mostly acute conditions (recent to one week) such as an accident or trauma.

NOTES:

Dog Acupuncture Points

Since there are hundreds of acupuncture points in the body, we are going to concentrate on just a few of them. You can then take the knowledge of using tuning forks and extend it to using them on the other acupuncture points for any animal.

We will be focusing on the following 10 points:

1-Shanken

2-Tienmen (Fengfu)

3-Sanjiang

4-Erhchien

5-Chingmei

6-Tachui

7-Weijian

8-Shenshu

9-Waikuan

10-Huantiao

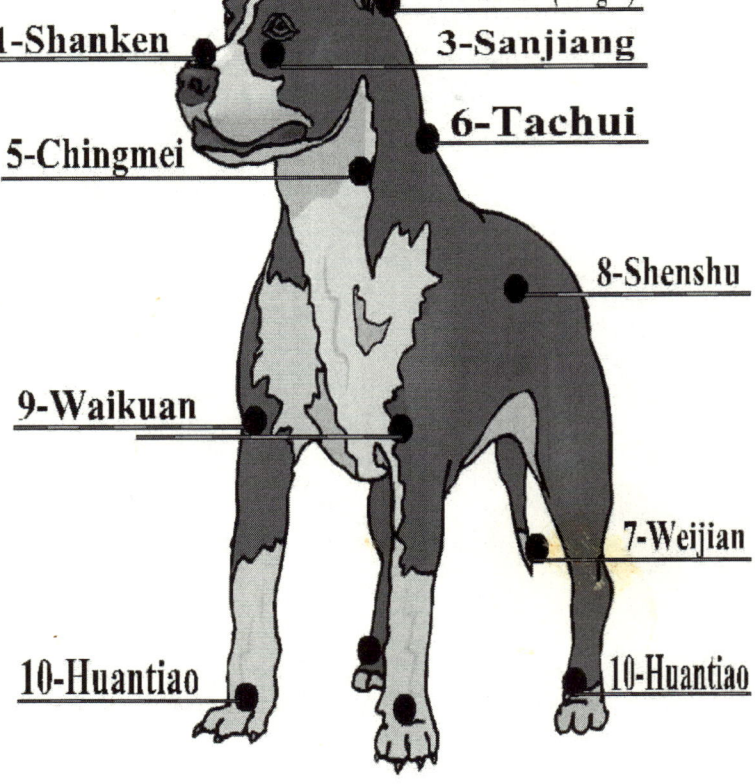

4-Erhchien-Tip of Auricle

2-Tienmen (Fengfu)

1-Shanken

3-Sanjiang

6-Tachui

5-Chingmei

8-Shenshu

9-Waikuan

7-Weijian

10-Huantiao

10-Huantiao

The first association we will make with the 10 acupuncture points is with their corresponding tuning forks using the Harmonic set of tuning forks.

This association is as follows:

1. **Shanken - tuning fork A**
2. **Tienmen -tuning fork B**
3. **Sanjiang - tuning fork Middle C & A**
4. **Erhchien - tuning fork B**
5. **Chingmeiv- tuning fork F**
6. **Tachui - tuning fork F**
7. **Weijian - tuning fork Middle C**
8. **Shenshu - tuning fork D**
9. **Waikuan - tuning fork Middle C and D**
10   **Huantiao - tuning fork Middle C**

1-Shanken

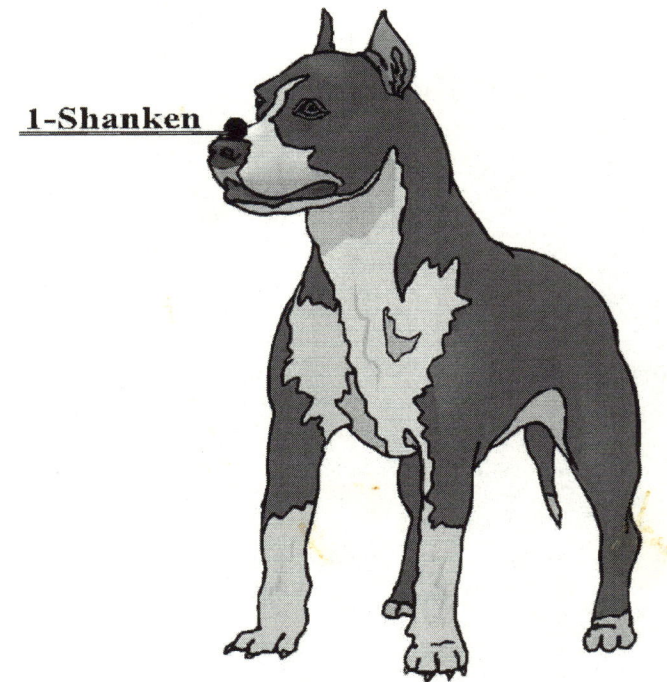

1-Shanken

Shanken is located over the nose at the midpoint connecting the inner canthuses of the eyes. This point borders the haired and the hairless parts.

Use this point for:

> **Apoplexy**
>
> **Heat-Stroke**
>
> **Sinus/Common cold**
>
> **First symptoms of febrile diseases**

Another point that is extremely well known is the **Su Liao**, or **GV 25** acupuncture point. The English name of this point is "White Bone-Hole." It is located on the tip of the nose and lies on the Governing Vessel Meridian. Please, do <u>not</u> use Moxa on this point as it is very sensitive and delicate.
*

Use this Point to:

- **Restore consciousness**

- **Maintain consciousness**

- **Shock**

- **Loss of consciousness**

- **Revive from drowning**

- **Rosaccea**

- **Nasal ailments (polyps, discharge, rhinitis)**

- **Olfactory changes (becomes sensitive to smells and aromas, lack of smell)**

- **Reduce alcohol intoxication from accidental ingestion of alcohol**

There are 28 Governing Vessel Meridian Points in all.

2-Tienmen (Fengu)

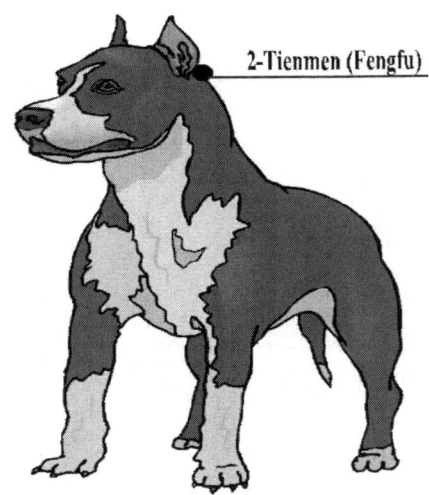

2-Tienmen (Fengfu)

       Tienmen is located at the top of the head at a midpoint of the horizontal line below the occiput. To locate this point, find the bottom of your dogs skull (occipitual bone) and find the center of that line with the top of your pet's head.

Use this point for:

> **Epilepsy**
>
> **Febrile diseases**
>
> **Encerphalitis**
>
> **Convulsion**
>
> **Limb spasms**

       This is the GV16 acupuncture point whose Chinese name is **'Feng Fu'** meaning **Wind Mansion** in English. It is located 1 cun directly above the midpoint of the PHL, directly below the occipital protuberance on the posterior midline of the head.

This point is the intersecting Point of the Governing Vessel, Yang Wei Vessel & Urinary Bladder Channel

Do not use Moxa and do not do Deep Needling on this point

Use this point to help:

- **Relieve headaches due to colds**
- **Relieves stiff neck**
- **Aversion to wind**
- **Dizziness (head)** and/or **(vision)**
- **Numbness**
- **Twitching (nervous conditions), Tremors**
- **Promotes communication between the mind and body**
- **Throat issues (swlling)**
- **Nosebleeds**
- **Earaches**
- **Eye pain**
- **Aphasia**

-On an emotional level, this point helps with fear, fright, and mania

-Main point for exterior and interior wind conditions.

3-Sanjiang

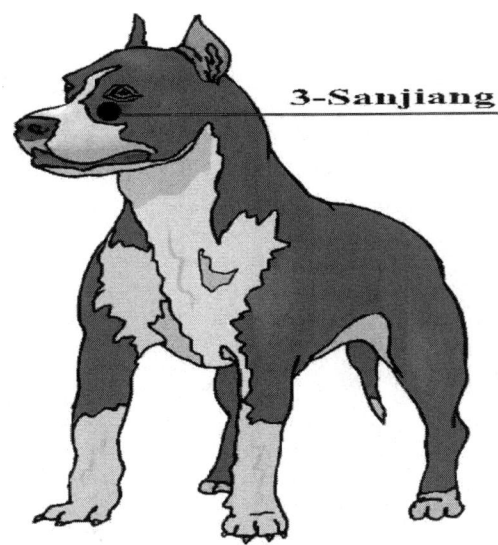

Locate this point just below your pet's eyes on the canthus vein at the inner canthuses. There is a point under the right and left eye.

Use this point for:

      Constipation, Diarrhea

      Abdominal pains

      Conjunctivitis

      Expels wind and heat from the throat, teeth, mouth, face and eyes

This is the **LI3** Acupuncture point and in one Chinese translation it is called **San Jian**. In English, it known as the **Third Space**. This point is located along the Large Intestine Meridian where there are 20 points in all.

4-Erhchien

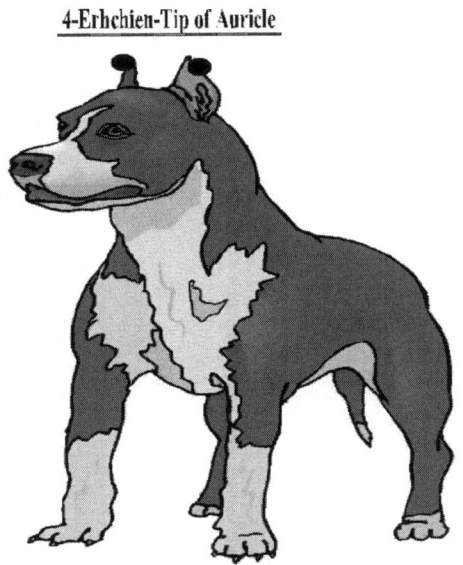

4-Erhchien-Tip of Auricle

Locate this point on the posterior (outer) tips of the auricles (ears). There is a point on both the right ear and the left ear.

Use this point for:

>**Apoplexy**
>
>**Heat-Stroke**
>
>**Herniary ache**
>
>**Convulsion**
>
>**Common cold**
>
>**Conjunctivitis**

This is the **LI2** acupuncture point. It lies on the Large Intestine Meridian to which there are 20 points.

There are many versions for the Chinese name of this acupuncture point. One such name that is used is called the **'Er Jian,'** in English it means **'Second Space.'** Another name for this point in Chinese is **'Ergian'**, which in English means **'Ear Apex.'** This one is more appropriate for our use as we will be activating the point on the very tip of the ear (the ear apex).

Use this point to:

- Hypertension

- To increase saliva production. Useful for dry mouth (xerostomia)

- Treats excess and clears heat from opposite end of the channel

- Toothache

- Eye redness

- Eye pain

- Gum inflammation

- Sore Throat

This point is usually bled to reduce strong heat in the body - high fever, red/swollen throat, mumps, etc.

5-Chingmei

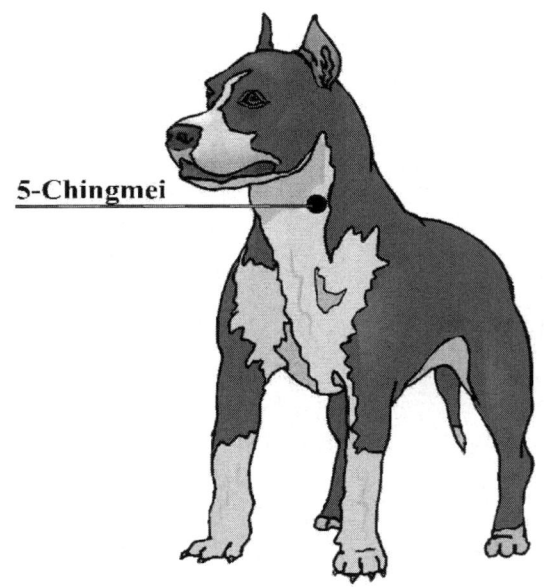

5-Chingmei

You can locate this point by following the venae cervicalis externus about one third of the way down the neck. This point includes the scapular muscle in the upper area and the superior thoracic muscle in the lower area.

Use this point for:

       Pneumonia

       Toxic effect

       Heat-Stroke

6-Tachui

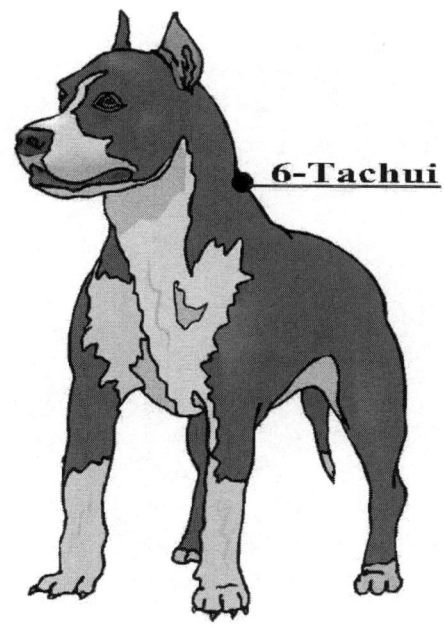

6-Tachui

This point is located in the depression between the spinous process between the first and the second thoracic vertebra. It is the GV13 and is located on the Governing Vessel Meridian.

Use this point for:

        Fever, Tonic

        Neuralgia. Rheumatism

        Bronchitis, Cough, Asthma

        Epilepsy. Traumatism

        Tonic

7-Weijian

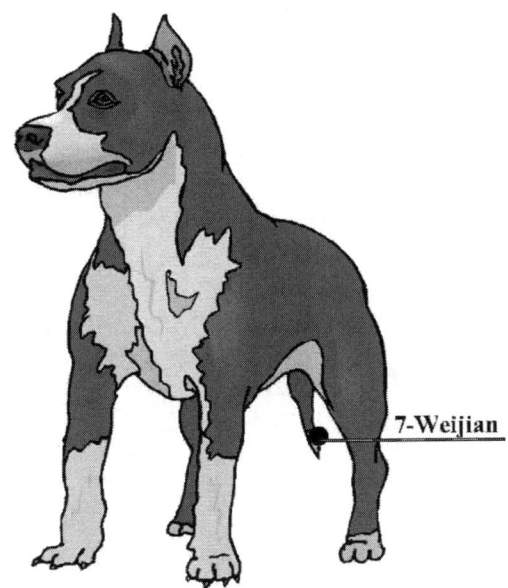

This point is located at the coccygeal end/nerve of the tail.

Tip of Tail

Use this point for:

        Apoplexy

        Heat-Stroke

        Gastroenteritis

The next closet point is the **GV 1** acupuncture point that is known at **'Chang Qiang'** in Chinese and **'Long Strong'** in English. It is located midway between the tip of the coccyx bone and the anus.

This is the intersecting Point of the Governing Vessel, Conception Vessel, Kidney & Gall Bladder Channels

Use this point for:

• **hemorrhoids from excess or deficiency (anal fissure, anal prolapse)**

• **diarrhea (without blood in the stools)**

• **constipations**

• **genitourinary disorders**

• **urinary retention**

• **sexual exhaustion**

• **impotence**

• **seminal emission**

• **disorders (and injuries) of the coccyx**

• **epilepsy**

• **manic depression**

8-Shenshu

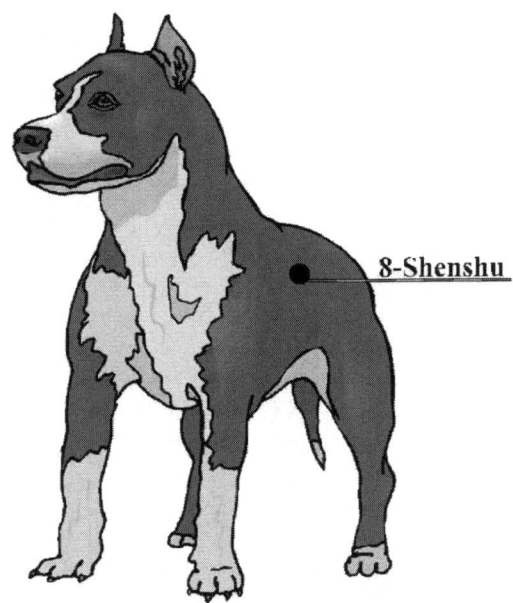

This point is located midway between the ilium and the last rib of the musculature and opposite of the horizontal protrusion of the 2nd lumbar vertebrae on both sides of the body.

Use this point for:

        Nephritis

        Urinary problems including excess urination

        Sexual Gland/Sterility/Impotence

        Lumbar Rheumatism and/or Muscle sprain

This is the **BL23** acupuncture point that is located on the Bladder Meridian.

Known by the Chinese name, **'Shen Shu,'** it is translated in English meaning, **'Kidney Shu.'**

Use this point for:

- Kidney issues and ailments

- Impotence

- Sterility

- Amenorrhea

- Infertility

- Low Back Pain

- Sprains

- Strains

- Tonify exhaustion and weakness

- Chronic Fatigue

- Ear problems (tinnitus, deafness, ear infrections)

There are 67 acupuncture points in the Bladder Meridian

9-Waikuan

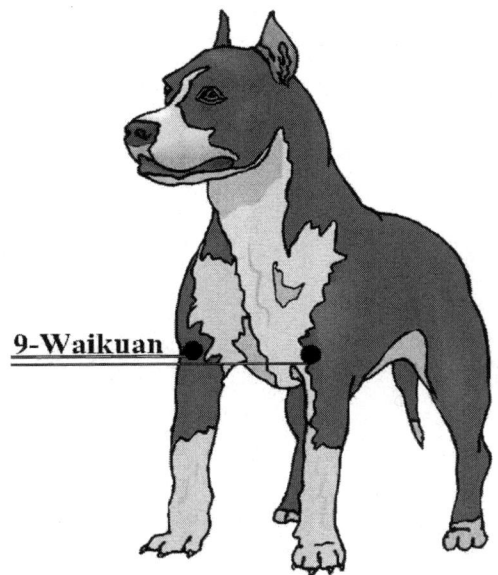

9-Waikuan

Located on the outer side of the front legs, this point is approximately ¼ of the length from the top of the leg. The point lies in a cavity between the ulna and the radius (the two bones of the front leg which are easily palpitated.)

This is the **TH5** acupuncture point and it is located along the Triple Heater Meridian. The point is called **'Waiguan'** in Chinese and **'Outer Pass'** in English. There are 23 points on this Meridian.

Use this point for:

- **Headaches, migraines**
- **Tonify for wind-cold, cold-damp**
- **Sedate for wind-heat (fever)**
- **Neck Stiffness**
- **Upper limb disorders** (elbow, forearm, wrist and hand)
- **Alternating fever and chills**
- **Leg problems**
- **Constipation**
- **Insufficient milk**
- **Paralysis of radial or ulnar nerve**
- **Rheumatism**

10-Huantiao

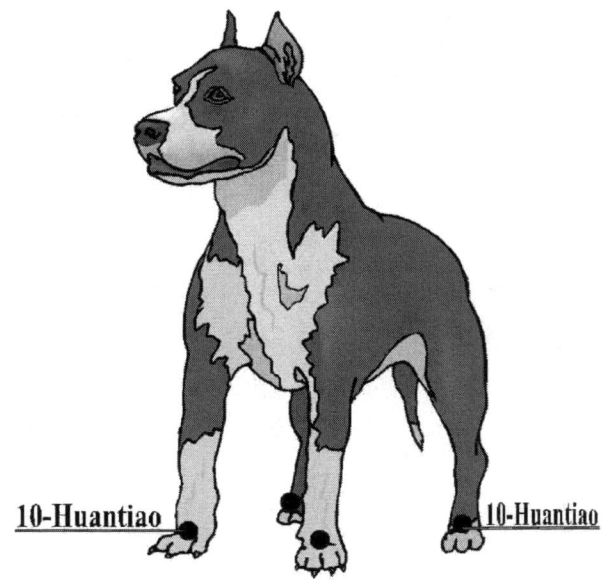

10-Huantiao   10-Huantiao

These points are located on the posterior(outer)-superior (top) side of the greater trochanter of the femur bone. There are 4 points in all.

Use this point for:

- **Sciatica**

- **Femoris Neuroparalysis**

- **Paralysis of the hind trunk**

- **Paralysis of the pelvis nerve branch**

- **Neuralgia of the pelvis nerve branch**

This is the **GB30** acupuncture point and is located on the Gall Bladder Meridian. There are 44 points along this Meridian.

This point is known by the Chinese name, **'Huan Tiao,'** and translated into English it means, **'Jumping Round.'**

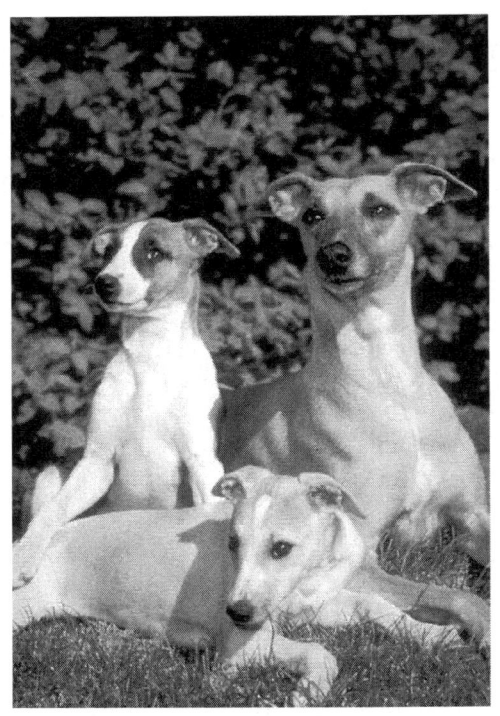

Chapter Ten

Ways to Select your Tuning Forks

How can I determine which tuning fork to use?

There are many ways in which you can select which tuning fork, or forks, to use and over which part of the body to use them.

1. Kinesiology

This is the simplest way to select the fork, or forks you are going to use in a healing session: You just ask! (Yes, you are asking your higher self).

2. The Five Element Theory

You can also select the forks you are going to use based on the symptomatic pattern of the pet's problem. Thus, if a pet is suffering with digestive problems, you will select the forks associated with the stomach/liver/gallbladder/small intestine and spleen/pancreas meridian. More on this in future Tuning Fork levels of study.

3. Dowsing

You may select the forks that are required for the pet by dowsing them together with the required area. Through dowsing, you can also ask for direction for treatment on the body and in the aura.

4. Relationship

Pain areas can be related back to the nearest Meridian circuits passing through the area or the nearest Chakra. You could then use the fork associated with that Chakra.

Tuning Fork Methods and Techniques

- **The Direct Contact Technique**
- **The Spiral Technique**
- **The Horizontal Technique**

The Direct Contact Technique

In the Direct Contact Technique you place the vibrating tip of the chosen tuning fork directly on the point selected. You will hold the vibrating tuning fork on the point for approximately 10 seconds and then you will reactivate the tuning fork and perform the technique again in the same spot for a total of three repetitions before moving on to the next point. If desired, and if you pet is willing, you can stay on a point for more than three repetitions.

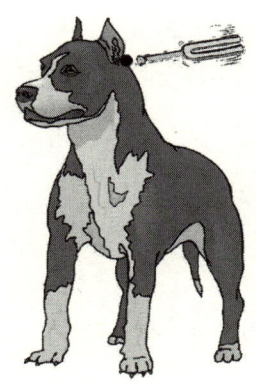

The Spiral Technique

Tuning forks can be used in a spiral pattern in three different ways. You may start at a specific location and begin making large, spiraling circles that get smaller as you lift the fork up from the body. I lift the fork to about 10" to 12" off the body. I normally perform these circles in a clockwise fashion. This will *open* closed chakras.

You may start with small spiraling circles that become larger and larger as you raise the tuning fork higher and higher away from the body. I usually perform this one in a counter clockwise fashion. This will *activate* and *energize* the chakra.

The third way is to make large spiraling circles about 12" above the body. As you slowly lower the tuning fork, you are also making the spiral smaller and smaller until you eventually end at a chakra point on the body. I normally do this pattern in a clockwise fashion to *sedate* and *calm* an over-active chakra.

NOTE: You may use the spiral technique if you need to 'open' your pet's chakra before treatment. I like to perform the spiral technique first on ALL of the chakras at least one time before I begin to use the direct contact technique on the pet. I then finish with the horizontal technique. You will find more information on this in my book on using tuning forks on dog's chakras.

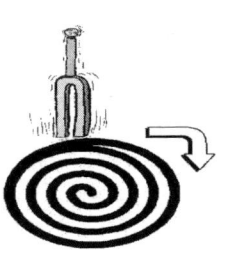

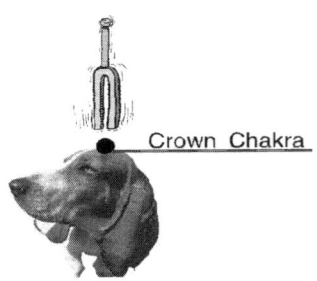

Crown Chakra

Horizontal Technique

In this technique you will place the vibrating tuning fork over the selected area of the body. Strike the tuning fork and, beginning on one side of your pet, pass the vibrating tuning fork 1"24" above the physical body to the other side and back again.

Count to 20 seconds while doing this technique. Shake off the fork, strike it again, and repeat the above process for a total of three sets of complete passes.

I generally start at the root chakra, move on to the sacral chakra, the solar plexus chakra, the heart chakra, the throat chakra, the brow chakra, the crown chakra, the soul start chakra, and then return to the earth star chakra to finish this technique. I use the corresponding tuning fork for each chakra.

In my sessions, I use the Spiral Technique to open chakras and energy centers, the Direct Technique to work on specific points and areas in need, and then I use the Horizontal Technique to balance the energy and close the energetic body and chakra system.

When finished with the session, I will then close the session using one of the closing techniques which will be discussed a little later in the book.

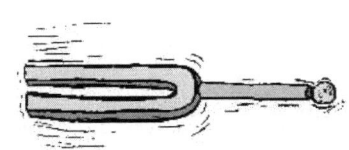

Crown Chakra

Aura-Smoothing Technique (closing)

There are many ways to complete your session with your pet and they may, or may not, include the use of tuning forks. Below is a list of some of the techniques. The more you work with energy the more you will discover new and inventive ways to perform the session.

Not one way is right and not one way is wrong. You must use your intuition to create the best possible environment and intention for you and the pet.

Using Tuning Forks on your Pet

1.   With both of your hands, gently use your fingers like teeth of a comb and "comb" through your pet's aura at about 4"-6" above the physical body.

2.   You can also use your hands to smooth out the aura by imitating "petting a dog." Just start at the head of the dog, about 4"-6" above the physical body, and "pet" the aura down to the dog's tail. Do this several times until you can feel the aura is smoothed out and free flowing. Yes, you can actually feel "bumps," "dips," and "valleys" in the aura.

3.   Another great way to end the session would be to give your pet a loving massage. Begin at your pet's face and with your hands on either side of your pet's face, run your hands down both sides of your pet to their tail. Do this three times trying to take in as much area as possible.

When I use tuning forks in my session, I activate either the 'C' 256 Hz, or use the OM tuning fork. I make three passes down the animal. The first pass begins on the animal's left side from about 10" to 12" above their head to down by their paws and back up again. The second pass is on the animal's right side starting from over their head to down by their paws and back up again. And the third pass begins over the animal's head in the center of their body to down by their paws and back up again.

Make sure that you shake your tuning fork off after each pass and that you reactivate your tuning fork when you moving in a new direction. You can use this technique in the same way for your pet.

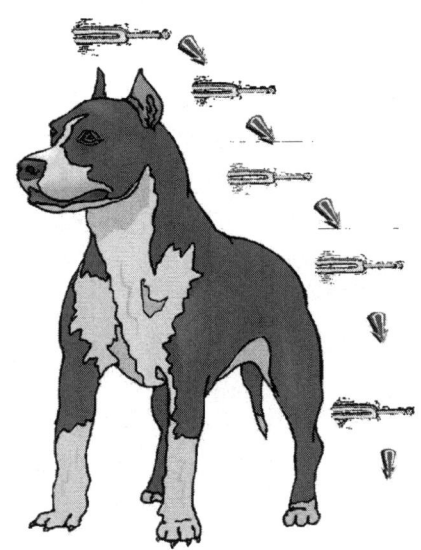

The Tuning Fork Therapy® Pet Session

There are many ways to go about giving your pet a Tuning Fork Therapy® session. You can either do a complete session, or a spot treatment for specific issues. A complete session would look as follows:

#1-How to Perform a Tuning Fork Therapy® Pet Session
(Specific Version)

1.   Take an animal health history.
2.   Decide what tuning forks you will need to work with.
3.   Center and ground yourself.
4.   Perform the Spiral Technique to **Open** energy centers.
5.   Go directly to the 'area' or 'condition' that the animal is suffering from and use the specific tuning fork designated for that area or condition. This is the Direct Contact Technique. Continue using forks on these areas until you can 'intuit' that you have done enough, or when the animal has signaled to you that it has had enough. Animals will tell you when they have had enough sound and vibrational energy - unless they are too ill to communicate to you. **(Tones and Balances)**
6.   Use the Horizontal Technique making 3 passes over the area or condition in question. **(CLOSES)**
7.   Follow with the Aura-Smoothing Technique. You can repeat this session several times throughout the day as needed.

Musical Terms Glossary

Amplitude-Another work for amplitude is loudness. The amplitude corresponds to how much the wave is compressed. It is also known as the pressure amplitude.

Chords—Chords are groups of three or more notes played, or sung, simultaneously. Each chord has a distinctive sound. The notes of a chord can be played all at once or one at a time. Every chord is built on a pitch, called the root. The sound of the chord depends on the intervals between the root and the other notes of the chord. Example: C major, F Minor, etc

Decibel-A decibel is the common measurement of loudness. It can be written out as decibel (dB). It is 1/10 of a bel, (named after the inventor of the telephone, Alexander Graham Bell).

Frequency-**The frequency of sound is the rate at which an object vibrates. It is also the rate at which the sound waves pass a given point. Frequency is also referred to as the pitch of a sound, or the note in musical sounds.**

Hertz (HZ)—**the n**umber of cycles per second.

Interval—an interval is the distance between two pitches. They are measured in terms of C major notes. To attain the interval, you count the distance in the alphabet between the two notes, including the notes. For example: the interval between Middle C and the G above it is a fifth: c/1, d/2, e/3, f/4, and g/5.

Meter—Meter is the repeating pattern of beats. The meter can be a grouping of any number of beats, but the human brain can't handle numbers past 13.

Note—in common usage, we refer to the note as the pitch, and it is also a symbol for a pitch. Notes appear on the music sheet as black dots, which symbolize pitch (duration).

Pitch—The pitch or note of a sound is determined by its wavelength/frequency. The shorter the wavelength/higher the frequency, the higher the pitch that we hear.

Relationship-The relationship between velocity, wavelength and frequency is: **velocity = wavelength x frequency**

Rhythm—Rhythm is the placement of sounds in time. This placement occurs in patterns. Usually, it appears in a repeating format. Rhythm can be further broken down into beats or pulses. In aerobics, instructors learn to hear this beat (usually an 8 count) and use this to smoothly change and transition into another exercise movement.

Scales and Keys—A scale is the definite internal relational structure with a "home" pitch; the note a melody usually ends on so that it sounds complete. A key is the tonal environment of a particular melody or scale.

Speed-**Speed is also known as the velocity of sound. The speed of sound in air is approximately 344 meters/second, 1130 feet/sec. or 770 miles per hour at room temperature of 20°C (70°F).**

Timbre—Pronounced (tam-ber). It is the quality that makes the Middle C of a piano sound different than the Middle C of a flute. Differences in timbre are the result of variations in the strength and tuning of the various overtones.

Triads—Triads are the simplest kind of chord as it consists of only three notes. The sound of a triad differs depending on the intervals between the notes. (The most common triads are the majors and minors.)

Velocity-Although Velocity is sometime referred as speed, there is a difference. Velocity includes the direction in which sound travels. Speed does not.

Wavelength-**Wavelength is the distance from one crest, or hump, of a wave to another crest, or hump, of the wave.**

About the Author

Francine Milford, LMT, Reiki Master
Reiki Center of Venice
P.O. Box 554, Venice, FL 34284-0554
www.ReikiCenterofVenice.com

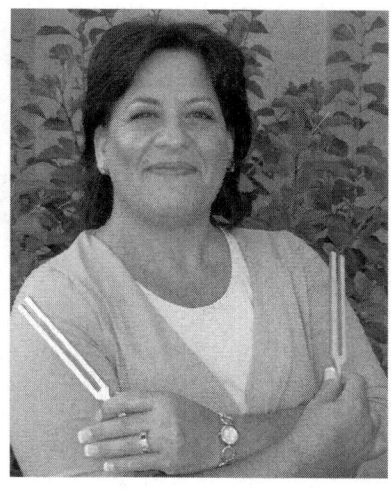

Francine Milford is a Holistic Practitioner, a national and state licensed massage therapist, personal trainer and owner of the Reiki Center of Venice. Francine created the Reiki Center of Venice, School of Massage Therapy and Bodywork where she educated others in a host of alternative therapies. She is an inspirational teacher and continuing education provider for many National Certifying Boards.

Francine Milford has attained Reiki Mastership through several lineages and brings her combined knowledge of energy work into her classes. *"Reiki has changed my life and has helped me to evolve on my Spiritual journey. It is the single best thing, next to Tuning Fork Therapy® that I have done for myself,"* said Francine.

Having experience in the Fitness Industry as a Personal Trainer and Aerobic Instructor, she has created a series of workshops and classes that combine the Body, the Mind, and the Spirit.

Francine offers a warm "can do" attitude in relating her own story of healing from debilitating and blinding migraines and constant panic attacks.

Through combining breathing techniques, relaxation techniques, tuning forks and exercise, along with Reiki, Francine has been symptom free for over five years.

It was during this time that Francine discovered her severe reactions to chemical drugs that were first prescribed to her by conventional doctors. "I didn't want to live like a zombie, dependent on pills. I wanted my health back and I began to search for the answers." Her search led her to study Herbology, Aromatherapy, Acupressure, Reflexology, and others forms of Alternative Therapy.

After several years of study and practicing various methods and techniques, Reiki was the icing on the cake. Francine now teaches courses in Alternative Therapies, both on site and by correspondence courses. Students can work at their own pace, one lesson at a time.

"Music has always been a part of my life and has affected me in many ways. I have played the piano since the age of 7. Later, I tried my hand at the clarinet, guitar, flute, and drums.

When tuning forks were first offered on the market, I was immediately drawn to them and the beautiful crystal resonance they provide. It wasn't until years later that I began to use tuning forks in my healing sessions for others.

By combining my knowledge, I have been able to create the Tuning Fork Therapy® series of books, manuals and certifications.

And I am hardly finished in learning additional systems of healing. *With every new system of healing, there is something I can take away and incorporate into my own practice. Learning never ends and I am enjoying the journey."*

You can view some of my courses, workshops and class schedules on my websites at:

www.ReikiCenterofVenice.com

www.TuningForkTherapy.com

Other Book Titles by this Author

Tuning Fork Therapy® Levels One through Eight

Tuning Fork Therapy®: Using Tuning Forks in Water

Tuning Fork Therapy® and High Blood Pressure

Tuning Fork Therapy®: How to Make a Gem Elixir

Tuning Fork Therapy®: How to use Planetary Tuning Forks

Assessing your Body's Energy System

Usui Reiki Level One Manual, Level Two Manual, Master Manual

Hand Therapy for Computer User

Makko Ho: Six simple exercises for Health and Vitality

DoIn: A form of self massage

The Basics of Sprouts

H2O Workouts: Basic Moves

H2O Workouts: Using your Pool Noodle

Vibrational Reiki™ Series of books and certification

Aroma~Care Books™: How to Make a Magical Blend

Aroma~Care Books™: How to Make a Perfume

Aroma~Care Books™: Pet Aromatherapy

Tuning Fork Therapy®: Using Tuning Forks on Dogs Chakras

Tuning Fork Therapy®: Using Tuning Forks on Cats Chakras

See the latest book titles at www.lulu.com/Francine

References:

1. **American Journal of AP** (1973-), Quarterly Journal.

2. **Scandinavian Journal of AP and Electrotherapy**, from Pekka Pontinen, 4-B-77 Pikkusaarenkuja, Tampere, Finland.

3. Anonymous (1993) Academy of Traditional Medicine, Beijing. **Essentials of Chinese AP**. English version. Foreign Languages Press, Beijing 432pp.

4. Anonymous (1977a) United States Dept. **Health translation of official Chinese (1970) manual. A barefoot doctor's manual**. Running Press, 38 South 19th St., Philadelphia, Pennsylvania, USA 948pp.

5. Brunner, F. (1980) **Akupunktur der Kleintiere**. WBV Biologisch Med. Verlag, Ipweg 5, D7060 Schorndorf, Germany 309pp.

6. Gilchrist, D. (1981) **Manual of AP for small animals**. PO Box 303, Redcliffe, Queensland 4020, Australia 79pp.

7. Klide, A.M. and Kung, S.H. (1977). **Veterinary AP**. University of Pennsylvania Press, Philadelphia, Pennsylvania USA 297pp.

8. Lin, J.H. and Rogers, P.A.M. (1980). **AP effects on the body's defense system: a veterinary review**. Veterinary Bulletin (August issue), 50, 633-640.

9. O'Connor, J. and Bensky, D. (1975) **Summary of research on the effects of AP**. American Journal of Chinese Medicine, 3, 377-394.

10. Rogers, P.A.M. and Bossy, J. (1981) **Activation of the defense systems of the body in animals and man by AP and moxibustion: additional evidence from the Peking** (1979) Symposium: AP Research Quarterly (Taiwan), 5, 47-54.

11. Rogers, P.A.M. (1990) **AP for immune-mediated disorders**. Chapter 14 of text on Veterinary AP. Lippincott Publishers, USA, in press.

12. Goldman, Jonathan, *Healing Sounds*. Element Books. Shaftesbury, ISBN 1-85230-314-X. 1992.

13. Tomatis, Alfred. *The Conscious Ear*. Station Hill Press. New York. ISBN 0-88268-108-7. 1991.

14. Maman Fabien. *The Role of Music in the Twenty-First Century*. Tama-Do Press. California. P61. ISBN 0-9657714-0-7. 1997.

15. Campbell, Don. *The Mozart Effect*. Avon Books. New York. ISBN 0-380-97418-5. 1997.

16. Emoto Masaru. *The Message from Water*. HADO Kyoikusha. Tokyo. ISBN 4-939098-00-1. 1999.

17. Davis, Audrey B. and Merzbach, Uta C. Early Auditory Studies: Activities in the Psychology Laboratories of American Universities. Washington: Smithsonian. (1975).

18. Miller, D. C. An Anecdotal History of the Science of Sound: To the Beginning of the 20th Century. New York: MacMillan. (1935).

19. A Handbook of Acupuncture Treatment for Dogs and Cats compiled by Lee-kin and translated by Tin-shen., Published & Printed in Hong Kong. Medicine & Health Publishing Co.

Websites:

Tuning Fork Therapy® homepage - www.TuningForkTherapy.com

http://www.vetmed.wsu.edu/ClientED/anatomy/

Made in the USA
Middletown, DE
21 February 2016